Understanding Pregnancy Loss

Also by Christine Moulder

Miscarriage: Women's Experiences and Needs 2nd edn (1995)

Understanding Pregnancy Loss
Perspectives and issues in care

Christine Moulder

MACMILLAN

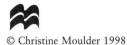

© Christine Moulder 1998

First published 1998 by
MACMILLAN PRESS LTD
Houndmills, Basingstoke, Hampshire RG21 6XS
and London
Companies and representatives
throughout the world

ISBN 0–333–72145–4 paperback ✓

A catalogue record for this book is available
from the British Library.

This book is printed on paper suitable for recycling and
made from fully managed and sustained forest sources.

10 9 8 7 6 5 4 3 2 1
07 06 05 04 03 02 01 00 99 98

Editing and origination by
Aardvark Editorial, Mendham, Suffolk

Printed in Malaysia

Contents

List of Tables

Foreword

I am delighted to write the preface for this book, which I believe breaks new ground in its treatment of the subject of pregnancy loss. As the author says, attitudes to pregnancy loss and technological developments have changed women's expectations, increased knowledge and fundamentally altered professional practice in the last twenty years.

The author's study of twenty women, each of whom had undergone pregnancy loss, whether stillbirth, miscarriage or termination of pregnancy, paints a moving picture of their feelings, experiences, the way they viewed their care from health professionals and their image of the health services provided in their southern England locality.

These women identified 70 health professionals who provided significant care to them. Interviews with these professionals brought out their views and attitudes to pregnancy loss, their practice, their feelings of adequacy and other constraints on caring for women in this situation.

The book points up vividly how women's experiences vary according to local professional or administrative policy, geographical constraints, fragmentation of care and, not least, the woman's own expectations both of the pregnancy and the circumstances of its loss, within her personal life.

I recommend this book to all health professionals who care for women undergoing pregnancy loss, involuntary or voluntary, wherever they need care – in hospital or in the community. Women in this situation need excellent clinical care, appropriate support and counselling on an individual basis, within a health care setting which is sensitively and sympathetically organised.

This book will help health professionals and interested others to reconsider their own attitudes to pregnancy loss, to examine their professional practice and to relook at the organisation of the service in which care to women is being offered.

Joan Greenwood OBE BA RGN RM MTD
July 1997

Preface

This project grew out of my membership of the national working party which helped to develop the *Guidelines for Professionals: Miscarriage, Stillbirth and Neonatal Death* published by SANDS (Stillbirth and Neonatal Death Society) in 1991. It was evident that producing guidelines in itself would do little to change policy and practice and that the recommendations made in the *Guidelines* made enormous demands on health professionals. Whilst there was a lot of anecdotal evidence there was little systematic research on women's experiences of health care or of health professionals' subjective experience of providing that care.

This study was designed to begin to fill that gap and to address the issues for professionals of the implementation of the policy and practice around pregnancy loss, as recommended in the SANDS *Guidelines*. The *Guidelines* defined the aspects of care to be investigated. A detailed case study approach was adopted which incorporated termination of pregnancy as well as stillbirth and miscarriage, but not neonatal death, and therefore challenged the traditional categorisation of pregnancy loss. The study is woman centred and embraces the differenct perspectives of patient and professional in a straightforward and open manner. Funding did not allow for the views of the women's partners to be sought.

The study is limited, undertaken in one hospital with a small group of women and the health professionals who cared for them but its value, I believe, lies within its limitations. The richness of the depth and detail of the material, the focus on individual experience and the overview that is given of women's experiences from the beginning to the end of their health care is its very strength. The emotional aspects of pregnancy loss which so often take second place in health care can be fully explored.

Christine Moulder
July 1997

Acknowledgements

Many people have helped to bring this project to fruition and I am grateful to them all. I am indebted most of all to the women who so willingly joined the study and shared their experiences but also to the health professionals who gave freely of their time in a spirit of openness and generosity. The research which forms the basis of this book was funded by the Department of Health and I am grateful for their financial support.

Janet Bell, the researcher for the first 15 months of the project, worked hard to help set up the study and recruit the participants. She undertook a significant amount of the interviewing. Her work in reviewing the literature on stillbirth and termination of pregnancy is drawn on in chapter 1. Amanda Spiers worked as the administrative secretary for the first two years of the project. She helped to make it all happen in an organised way. Her support and interest in the project were invaluable when mine was flagging. Fiona Chandler assisted in the analysis of the data on the health professionals. Abigail Smith helped to prepare the final manuscript.

I am indebted to my colleagues at the Centre for Social Policy and Social Work at the University of Sussex not only for giving the project a home but also for providing me with a supportive working environment, particularly when the going got tough. Without Hugh England's initial encouragement the project would never have got off the ground and I am grateful for his support in managing the project. Judith Harwin's encouragement and interest have made a vital difference in the later stages. Crescy Cannan and Jenny Clifton provided invaluable consultation. John Jacobs gave generously of his time for discussion, for reading draft material and in the preparation of the final manuscript. I am particularly indebted to him for his help with the section on the health professionals.

I am grateful to Joan Greenwood for her encouragement and advice when the project was a germ of an idea and to Kate Sallah for her enthusiasm and support as the project developed. Nancy Kohner has willingly shared her knowledge and discussions with her have always been stimulating and supportive.

The advisory group have also played their part and I appreciate their support. My thanks go to Vicki Allanach, Royal College of Nursing; Sue Botes, Health Visitors Association; Joanie Dimavicius, SATFA; Mary El-Rayes, SANDS; Catherine McCormick, Royal College of Midwives; Gill Mallinson; Professor Richard Vincent, Trafford Centre for Medical Research, University of Sussex; and Dr Luke Zander, UMDS. Hilary Thomas' (University of Surrey) advice on the design and methodology were invaluable. Ruth Bender Atik (Miscarriage Association) and John Hare (Hinchingbrooke Hospital) both made detailed and helpful comments on draft material. Gerry Smale (National Institute for Social Work) made time to share his experience of organising research and his understanding of organisational change.

I am also grateful to Richard Pemberton for putting up with my absorption with pregnancy loss. He helped me to develop my ideas about good emotional care and to put the issues raised by the research in a broader context.

Christine Moulder
June 1997

This work was commissioned by the Department of Health. The views expressed in this publication are those of the author and not necessarily those of the Department of Health.

Chapter 1

Changing attitudes, changing practice

■ Introduction

Attitudes to pregnancy loss have changed fundamentally in the past 20 years. The impetus for much of the change has been from women themselves, acting either as individuals or through the self-help organisations: the Miscarriage Association, the Stillbirth and Neonatal Death Society (SANDS) or Support Around Termination for Abnormality (SATFA). These organisations formed in the late 1970s and 80s and continue to play a vital role not only in raising public awareness of the issues and providing support for women but also in acting as a resource group for professionals and pressing for improvements in health care.

There are broader changes which underpin the changing ideas about pregnancy loss. Our attitude to death and our response to dying are less of a taboo. In our society in the late 1990s there is greater openness to facing the reality of death as well as to participation in the decision-making and the ritual connected with it. The role of women has changed dramatically and there is greater focus on women's issues. It is hardly surprising that along with these developments comes an increased openness to issues to do with pregnancy loss.

Technological change has also played its part. In general terms it has made anything seem possible and encouraged the view that problems can be solved, which perhaps makes a failed pregnancy harder to accept. The widespread use of ultrasound in early pregnancy has, for many women, made the baby a reality from a much earlier gestation and for some the loss is therefore much greater. The introduction of widespread prenatal screening has changed the experience of early pregnancy and more women now face the prospect of considering a termination of pregnancy. Some would argue that the greater availability of testing for abnormality can delay attachment and investment in the pregnancy until it is known that the baby is healthy (Rothman 1986).

The development in reproductive technology has revitalised scientific interest in early pregnancy. The progress in infertility treatments has increased knowledge about conception and the development of the embryo.

1

Complex and profound issues about the use of human embryos and the morality of conception outside the womb are raised. Central to these debates are differing views about when human life begins and the status of the embryo/fetus. These issues have been brought to public attention but also have prompted government intervention to control and regulate such activity (the Embryology and Human Fertilisation Act 1990).

There have been other changes in policy which have brought issues to do with pregnancy loss to the fore. For example, the Polkinghorne Committee (Polkinghorne 1989), set up to advise on the use of fetal tissue resulting from abortions, addressed two issues of direct relevance. Firstly, in stressing that the mother's consent was essential, the rights of the woman over her fetus were established. Secondly, in recommending 'the respectful disposal of the dead fetus', the issue of disposal was brought to the fore. These recommendations in turn lent support to those clamouring for change and improvements in practice.

The changes in the management of pregnancy loss have occurred within, and reflect, a more general shift in the balance of power between patients and the medical establishment. There is more opportunity for women to express their views. Women as patients now expect as of right information about themselves and their treatment. Cultural and religious differences are slowly being acknowledged, and generally there is a greater anticipation of partnership between patient and health service, patients' needs and wishes being accommodated where possible rather than there being acquiescence to a 'doctor knows best' rule.

Changing Childbirth, the government initiative to develop maternity services, although saying relatively little about pregnancy loss, enshrined the principle of woman-centred care and emphasised the importance of continuity of care, choice, the role of a lead professional and the involvement of users in planning services. It is in the area of maternity care that the principles of partnership in care have been developed and put into practice. Maternity care is now being used as an example of how to take forward these principles in other areas of the NHS.

However, the quality and character of care that is provided for pregnancy loss is influenced by the way in which the experience is construed. Increasingly, pregnancy loss is viewed as a continuum of experience but services are usually organised around the different categories of experience according to gestation and whether or not the loss was voluntary. The care that is provided for women who miscarry, those whose babies are stillborn and those who have a termination of pregnancy is qualitatively different. Yet it can be argued that these divisions are arbitrary, do not reflect women's own experience of the event and, in the way they determine the reactions of others and the care that is provided, can be actively unhelpful.

To put this study of pregnancy loss in context it is important to consider in more detail the background to current understanding. This chapter draws on the lay, professional and academic literature about pregnancy loss to give an overview of some of the issues that inform views of women's experiences and the care that is provided. Consideration is then given to the development of the SANDS *Guidelines,* which can be seen as a statement of current views on good practice and which this study was designed to underpin.

■ Stillbirth

❏ Exposing the problem

Over the past 25 years the silence around stillbirth has been slowly broken, largely by women speaking out about their experiences but also by professionals. Accounts from parents, published in the SANDS newsletter, describe in a powerful and moving way the impact of stillbirth and the grief that follows (see also Kohner and Henley 1991). Professionals who have personal experience of stillbirth also write about themselves in the professional journals (Harvey 1983; Mitchell 1988). There is an immediacy about these accounts that is very affecting. There are no accounts from parents who have not experienced the death as a loss and no evidence from parents that some do not grieve.

It is only the women's accounts that detail the entire experience. The professional literature tends to fragment the event into separate parts – diagnosis, genetic counselling, care in hospital, aftercare, practical information for staff and so on. For each woman the experience will be unique and a function of many factors that are beyond the actual stillbirth event. However, some of the dimensions of the experience which will vary between women can be identified: the circumstances of the diagnosis, the management of labour, the state of the baby and the longer-term emotional consequences.

In 1968 Bourne identified stillbirth as a 'professional blind spot'. He found that the GPs in his study were largely unable to describe the experiences of their patients who had had a stillbirth. Fifteen years later there was a growing public awareness that there was still an issue for women who found that neither society nor the health services appropriately acknowledged their loss (Rantzen 1983). This questioned a prevalent feeling that the emotional impact of stillbirth could be reduced by not dwelling on it and that seeing and commemorating the baby increased attachment and therefore made it all worse. This was reflected in the attitudes of health staff and the management of the event in hospital and can be seen as a rationale for care that enabled professionals to avoid contact with parents and babies that they themselves found distressing.

❑ Confirming the existence of grief

The subsequent literature has attempted to describe the nature of the experience in the short and long term and to confirm it as a bereavement process (Kennell *et al.* 1970; Wolff *et al.* 1970; Dunlop 1979; Bourne 1983; Stierman 1987). Parkes' model of bereavement processes is widely cited. Numbness and shock are described (Chez *et al.* 1982; Kirk 1984; Defrain *et al.* 1990). Denial that this is happening at all is common and leads to parents looking for any hint that this might not be true. Parents may misconstrue what they see and are told to fit with their preferred interpretation of a live baby. The failure to produce the hoped for and expected live birth leads to a sense of failure, inferiority, shame and guilt (Lewis and Page 1978; Bourne and Lewis 1984). The resultant low self-esteem makes it less likely that parents will be able to express their needs. There is a strong sense of being out of control. Anger is another powerful emotion that is likely to find expression against professionals, partners or God. Pervading all of this is an increasing sense of despair.

A range of mourning symptoms and behaviours has been identified in women post-stillbirth: being woken in the middle of the night by a baby crying (Chez *et al.* 1982) and feeling the baby kicking after the birth (Condon 1986); thoughts such as wondering if the baby is warm enough and comfortable in the grave (Davis *et al.* 1988; Defrain 1990). Fears of going mad are common and 28 per cent of women in one sample had suicidal thoughts (Defrain *et al.* 1990). In the longer term a tendency has been observed of the dead baby being idealised, which may have an adverse effect on subsequent children who never live up to the ideal (Lewis and Page 1978).

Pathological grief has been identified as taking two forms – chronic, intense grieving and delayed or absent grieving (Leff 1987). Knowledge of these conditions is incomplete, but a link has been suggested between poor patient satisfaction with care, lower self-esteem and few memories of the baby, and severity of depression (Murray and Callan 1988). Much of the discussion about pathological reactions comes from psychiatrists who see only those whose response is considered pathological.

However, stillbirth is a complex and sensitive issue to research. Studies are often based on small, self-selected samples. Long-term follow-up studies are rare and the attrition rate is high. Measuring grief in any systematic way is also problematic. It is therefore difficult to describe the parameters of a 'normal' grief reaction following stillbirth, but six to nine months has been suggested (Condon 1986). It is reasonable to assume that resolution of grief is a very individual thing. Indicators such as age of mother, gestation, supportiveness of marital relationship and previous mental health symptoms have been identified as factors significant in the recovery of women in the short term (Toedter *et al.* 1988) but a longitudinal study of women over the entire grief period is still lacking.

❏ Ideas about good care

Much of the stillbirth literature addresses what is known about good care around the time of the event. Poor practice has been identified as having a detrimental impact on the recovery of women (Estok and Lehman 1983; Kirk 1984). There is little empirical research into evaluating services and attempts at identifying indicators of 'success' can flounder (Lake *et al.* 1987). Instead, services are described, leaving readers to make their own judgement (Sherratt 1987; Tom-Johnson 1990).

The current literature summarises what is believed to be good practice (Hutti 1984, 1988b; Condon 1987; Davis *et al.* 1988; Wathen 1990). Great weight is afforded to anecdotal evidence (Chez *et al.* 1982; Morris 1988b) and case studies (Lewis 1976). Early recommendations have now been accepted as good care and in recent years there has been a remarkable consensus about what should be offered to parents, but with a great focus on hospital treatment immediately around the time of the birth. Much less is known of the nature and efficacy of good follow-up support beyond the maternity ward.

The themes identified in the health professional press are confirmed in parents' accounts and revolve around empowering parents, giving clear information, gaining parents' views and enabling them to make decisions about their care. The notion that mothers can be spared pain and grief by not being involved in the care of their baby is now dismissed. Good care involves both parents as much as possible with their baby. It also means prompting reluctant parents to become involved with their baby. Seeing the baby, holding it, washing and dressing it, cuddling it, naming it and showing it to significant others are all activities that acknowledge the loss and mark the beginning of the normal grief process. Activities that were once described as healthy but 'bizarre' (Lewis 1979) are no longer identified as a problem for professionals. The pendulum has perhaps swung the other way and concern has been expressed (Leon 1992a, b) that the professional response may be institutionalised, grief homogenised and parents pressurised into behaving in certain ways against their wishes.

❏ Implications for health professionals

The events during the 'crucial hours' preceding and following the death have been identified as most significant for the emotional outcome for women (Condon 1987). This puts the responsibility for women's mental well-being firmly with the obstetric team. It is not special attention from experts that women need but appropriate care from those who expect to be present around any birth. Clearly, a great deal is asked of staff whose usual work activity is concerned with the very different atmosphere of the live, healthy birth.

The lack of literature up until the late 1970s has been seen as a manifestation of the discomfort of doctors with the whole subject of stillbirth. A *Lancet* editorial (*Lancet* 1977) referred to it as the 'last taboo' and only by the mid-1980s was it 'beginning to come out of the closet' (Kirk 1984). Although the issue of the stress the whole incident places on doctors was raised early on in the debate (Smith 1977) the difficulties inherent in this work are not well understood. It has been suggested that both medical and nursing staff feel incompetent at stillbirths and tend to identify women's losses with their own, making it difficult to spend time with women in the acute stages of grief (Danville 1983), and that obstetricians must address their feelings of disappointment and failure if they are to be able to respond to parents (Davis *et al.* 1988). The issues for professionals are hinted at but as yet not fully explored.

■ Miscarriage: usually a loss but always a crisis

Miscarriage has been the 'hidden experience', a minor medical event, socially unrecognised and kept out of the public domain. No national statistics are collected and the incidence of miscarriage is difficult to calculate. It is estimated that around one in five recognised pregnancies ends in miscarriage before 20 weeks gestation and that the rate is higher if preclinical miscarriages are included (Smith 1988).

It is only from the 1990s that gynaecological textbooks, lay books on pregnancy and childbirth, and even books on the social and political aspects of maternity, have begun to recognise the significance of miscarriage. Neither has it been an area of interest to those concerned with health policy or even women's studies. Some suggestions can be made for this neglect: that little can be done to prevent miscarriage, that there is a the lack of attention given to women's experience in a man's world and that insight into the experience of miscarriage challenges an acceptance of abortion based on denying the humanity of the embryo.

❏ From a woman's point of view: the dimensions of the experience

The major source of information about women's experiences of miscarriage is the literature aimed at women (for example Borg and Lasker 1982; Oakley *et al.* 1984; Leroy 1988; Hey *et al.* 1989; Moulder 1990). Brief descriptive accounts of personal experience have also appeared in the professional press (for example Nash 1987; Fewster 1990; Leask 1991). It can be criticised for being unrepresentative, drawing only on the experience of women who care enough about what has happened to them to write or talk about their miscarriage. Nevertheless the extensive personal accounts and case histories provide a rich source of descriptive data. Certain dimensions of the experience can be identified: the realisation of the miscarriage, the physical process, the management of the miscarriage and level of medical intervention, the reactions of partner, family, friends and health

professionals, as well as psychological reactions and the process of assimi-
lating the experience and moving on possibly to another pregnancy.

The small-scale qualitative studies of Swanson-Kaufman (1983) and
Hutti (1986) also emphasise the importance of these dimensions although
the terms they use in describing categories of experience differ. Agreement
with this view is not directly stated in the wider professional and academic
literature but it is clear that there is no active dissent with this portrayal of
the dimensions of women's experiences.

Furthermore, clear themes emerge from an analysis of women's accounts
of their experience. There is often a marked contrast between women's views
of their experience and others' perceptions. Most of the women who have
contributed to this literature conceptualise their miscarriage as a significant
event, usually as a loss with accompanying grief and mourning, whilst others,
be they partners, family, friends, acquaintances or health professionals, may
not necessarily do so. Consequently, women report that it is often hard to
share their experience constructively and to receive appropriate support.

In addition there are reports of dissatisfaction with health care
throughout the lay, clinical, professional and academic literature. The issues
women perceive as important are staff attitudes, denial of the meaning of
the event, the insensitive use of language, the lack of information and
explanation, poor facilities and the lack of follow-up care. These themes are
echoed in the literature based on clinical experience (for example Herz
1983; Graves 1987; Stirtzinger and Robinson 1989). Cecil's research in
Northern Ireland (1994) confirms these views and attributes the poor
quality of care to a lack of appreciation among health professionals of the
significance of an early pregnancy loss. She suggests that poor communication and a lack of time contribute to misunderstandings.

❏ Establishing the reaction to miscarriage as grief

Implicit and unchallenged in the lay literature is the idea that women experience miscarriage as a loss so their feelings afterwards are of grief. Many
women clearly describe their feelings in these terms. Indeed, much of the lay
literature and earlier clinical literature (for example Corney and Horton
1974; Peppers and Knapp 1980; Stack 1980; Leppert and Pahlka 1984) sets
out to establish the normality of a grief reaction following miscarriage and
the similarity with patterns of grief at the loss of a loved one.

The unique features of grief after a miscarriage are focused on: the lack
of ritual, not knowing who or what is lost, the loss of role and future hopes,
the private nature of the loss, helplessness to prevent it, the loss of a part of
oneself, the lack of explanation and the consequent feelings of guilt and
anger. However, it is also clear that women react in different ways to miscarriage and that for many their reactions are ambivalent. For example, Seibel
and Graves (1980) reported that nearly one third of the women reported
positive feelings (feeling happy, lucky or relieved) when they miscarried

whilst over a half reported feelings of depression and anxiety. It cannot be assumed that every woman experiences a miscarriage as a loss.

❏ The incidence of distress and predicting outcome

Recent research concentrates on assessing the psychological and psychiatric consequences of miscarriage (Seibel and Graves 1980; Friedman and Gath 1989; Jackman *et al.* 1991; Neugebauer *et al.* 1992; Thapar and Thapar 1992; Cecil and Leslie 1993; Garel *et al.* 1993; Prettyman *et al.* 1993; Cordle and Prettyman 1994; Robinson *et al.* 1994). Study designs vary extensively. A range of measures is used to assess short-term symptoms of depression and anxiety and to establish psychiatric 'caseness'. Sample sizes are often small and non-participation and drop-out rates high. The results of these studies are inconsistent and difficult to compare. However, all the studies report a varying proportion of women experiencing some form of distress. In her comprehensive review of studies that utilise concurrent rather than retrospective assessments of emotional states Slade (1994) concludes that probably between one fifth and one half of women risk significant depressive symptoms within the first month after a miscarriage and many women experience significant anxiety symptoms.

Attempts to understand which women are most at risk of severe reactions have not been very successful. A variety of factors have been suggested as affecting outcome, for example depressive symptoms and previous psychiatric history (Friedman 1989), aspects of medical management (Jackman *et al.* 1991) and social support (Cordle and Prettyman 1994; Lasker and Toedter 1994).

Slade (1994) critically reviews the psychological literature summarising the factors that have been considered as influencing outcome. She concludes that previous contact with services for emotional problems is the only factor that appears to be consistently linked with increased emotional distress. The other demographic factors appear to be unrelated whilst the evidence on reproductive history and aspects of pregnancy is conflicting. She acknowledges that factors to do with the process of the miscarriage and the impact of health care have largely been ignored. It is these last categories that emerge in analysis of the descriptive literature as being important to women, along with social support, which does not form part of Slade's critique.

❏ The diversity of experience

The limitations in a quantitative approach to understanding a complex psychological and social experience become apparent. The constructs used and the measures employed derive from a psychiatric ideology and serve to define and categorise women's experiences in a way which ignores the individual nature of the personal response to the event. Seibel and Graves first suggested in 1980 that 'what it means to her' is the major influence on a woman's reactions. Lovell (1983b), in stressing the importance of women's subjective perceptions of the event, and Hutti (1986), emphasising the influence of cognitive representations on individual grief responses, echo this approach. More recently, Slade (1994) suggests that the predictive value of much of the psychological literature is disappointing because the personal construction of the event is ignored.

For example, whilst one woman who has not planned to be pregnant may be relieved when she miscarries, another may be overwhelmed with guilt and self-blame. For some women with a history of infertility a miscarriage can be construed as a positive event because it is evidence that conception can be achieved whilst for others it will be an even greater loss. It is the individual interpretation of the circumstances of the event that is the key to understanding how women experience a miscarriage.

A picture emerges of women who react very differently over varying periods of time. There is ample evidence in the descriptive literature (for example Oakley 1984; Moulder 1990) to support this view. Women describe how their grief peaks and then fades and that this happens more quickly for some women than others. Some women are able to express their feelings more freely at the time whilst others put their feelings 'on hold' until they are able to deal with them, their feelings are perhaps never fully expressed. Women describe how it takes time for their feelings to emerge, perhaps triggered by a particular event.

This variety of pattern of reaction, although not peculiar to miscarriage, may be a reflection of the lack of social definition of the experience. The lack of prescribed rules and rituals following miscarriage means that a woman has, as suggested by Cormell (1990), to work out exactly what she is experiencing and to negotiate her own path to get through the experience and reach a point of resolution and acceptance in the aftermath.

❏ Changing care for miscarriage

Whilst much of the research addresses issues of health care provision based on criticisms of the prevailing system of care there is little research on health professionals' views of caring for women who miscarry. The literature, as with stillbirth, considers the aspects of health care that are helpful to women. Again the focus is more on hospital care although the importance of the provision of follow-up care and of opportunities for counselling is often mentioned (Turner 1989).

Much of the focus, in the face of the hidden nature of miscarriage, is on explaining the nature of the experience to health professionals. Emphasis is on how to help women, the need to acknowledge the reality of the loss, giving information and explanation and educating parents on their likely reactions (Hutti 1984, 1988c; Symonds 1988; Iles 1989; Moulder 1990; Defrain 1991). The dilemmas posed by the different interpretations of the experience by women are rarely explored.

Changes in views about the significance of miscarriage are reflected in changes in some aspects of the provision of care. The increased availability of ultrasound scanning has, from a woman's point of view, revolutionised care. The 'put your feet up and wait and see' approach is no longer acceptable. The introduction in some hospitals of early pregnancy assessment or fetal viability clinics, which aim to give prompt diagnosis and treatment, have streamlined health care for some women. Specialist recurrent miscarriage clinics are an acknowledgement of the needs of these women and a recognition that recurrent miscarriage, at least, is a condition worthy of investigation and, in some cases, treatment. Changes in treatment for early miscarriage currently being researched, evacuation of retained products of conception (ERPC), medical management or wait and see what happens (Henshaw *et al.* 1993a, b; Nielson and Hahlin 1995) introduce alternative courses of action for women.

■ Termination of pregnancy

❏ The moral debate

Abortion is an issue about which many people feel passionately and standpoints are rigorously defended. The right for women to choose not to continue with a pregnancy has been hard won. When an abnormality is detected the termination of pregnancy is presented as the solution to the problem of genetic disease. There is a powerful lobby that objects to termination of pregnancy on religious and moral grounds, publishing documents and producing evidence of the damage to women of terminating pregnancies – but not backed by research. The public debate is kept alive in the press by reports on such issues as sex selection and the use of fetal eggs and, more recently, with selective termination following infertility treatment. There is an ongoing moral debate in the medical press about the relative position of abortion in the broader 'institutionalisation of killing' (Muller 1991) and a warning that abortion on grounds of sex is a precedent to eugenics that should remain illegal (Evans *et al.* 1991).

The antithetical way in which abortion is perceived is reflected in the literature. There is a clear distinction between abortion for reasons that are not related to the physical health of mother or fetus, and termination for fetal abnormality. The two groups are not usually written about together. Psychological processes are ignored and it is assumed that the motivation for termination makes it into two entirely different experiences. There are different physical experiences for women based on the gestation of the pregnancy which, by and large, coincide with the reason for the termination. Most early terminations are carried out by suction before 14 weeks and most terminations for abnormality are in the second trimester, when labour will normally be induced.

❏ Early termination of pregnancy

Women's views

Although first-trimester termination of pregnancy is experienced by a large number of women there is very little written by way of first-hand accounts. Women are not organised into support groups and there is no forum for them to discuss the issues that it raises. Books have started to appear in the lay press (Neustatter and Newson 1986; Davies 1991) that describe women's experiences of early termination and aim to provide information and support for women who find themselves in the situation of trying to make a decision or who want to reflect on their experience. This work is based on the authors' own experiences and the accounts of a self-selecting group of women who respond to articles in magazines.

There is a consensus that women experience termination as a much more complex decision than the polarised pro-life versus pro-choice debates would suggest. Early termination can be seen as the last taboo. It is as if, having asked for and obtained a termination, women are expected to be pleased and relieved and any admission of negative feelings interpreted as regret: women are not entitled to grieve (Neustatter and Newson 1986, Chapter 4). However, it is likely that for women the early termination of pregnancy will include the following dimensions: the reason for being pregnant, making the decision, the pressure of time, arranging the termination, the procedure, the aftermath and (usually) the lack of follow-up care.

Emphasis of the research into first-trimester termination of pregnancy

Most of the medical research carried out into first-trimester abortion is aimed at establishing whether or not the procedure does women any psychological harm. There is a preoccupation with looking for negative outcomes, including guilt. The volume of research into the impact of abortion on women would appear to be a reaction to the moral debate about its availability rather than concern generated by the actual incidence of psychological damage identified.

This is a very difficult and sensitive area to research. Quantitative studies have been critically reviewed (Rogers *et al.* 1989) and found to be lacking, although it is appealing to those who feel that it is easier to defend 'scientific' data, and qualitative studies are also largely methodologically flawed (Lazarus and Stern 1986). Common problems are of small self-selecting or biased samples, high drop-out rates, varying timescales post-abortion, choosing and using assessment instruments, interview bias and the lack of baseline information. Extremely biased research is still being reported. It remains very difficult to be confident of a causal relationship between the abortion and subsequent psychological states.

However, within these limitations there is a fairly consistent finding that abortion for the woman who wants it does not cause long-term psychological disturbance for the majority, although there is certainly a short-term impact (Lask 1975; Ashton 1980). This research has been comprehensively reviewed (Adler 1992; Zolese and Blacker 1992).

For the majority of women the main emotions post-termination are of relief and happiness (Osofsky and Osofsky 1972; Greer *et al.* 1976) even when, had their circumstances been different, they would have elected to continue with the pregnancy. Often the time prior to the termination is one of great distress that is essentially ended with the procurement of the termination (Adler 1992), and depression among women has been found to be greater before the operation (Dagg 1991). For pro-life groups there is an obvious gain to identifying a negative reaction peculiar to abortion, such as post-abortion syndrome but this is not substantiated by any academic research.

A small proportion of women, five per cent (Ashton 1980), do go on to develop 'enduring, severe psychiatric disturbance' and work has been carried out on trying to develop indicators that would predict for which women this is likely to be a problem (Lask 1975; Belsey *et al.* 1977; Shusterman 1979). The factors identified that would appear to be significant in predicting adverse response to abortion appear to be the level of ambivalence about the decision, the perceived supportiveness of the partner and significant others, and the degree of psychological stability before the event. Ambivalence about the decision has also been identified as an indicator of slower psychological recovery (Shusterman 1979; Ashton 1980).

More recently it has been suggested that, whilst mourning does occur after a minority of abortions, a 'simple crisis-reaction model' would be more appropriate (Zolese and Blacker 1992). This also has the effect of framing the abortion in its wider context of an unwanted pregnancy, which is often lost in the consideration of the impact of abortion. The woman is not, of course, the only person to be affected by the decision to abort. There is evidence that one in three women who are denied abortion go on to resent their babies (Pare and Raven 1970). Some relationships can be strengthened by the experience (Ashton 1980), whereas some that are less stable may come under great strain, but separations that occur six months after the event are unlikely to be permanent (White-van Mourik *et al.* 1992).

❏ Termination for abnormality

Women's views

Parents who have made the abortion decision after a diagnosis of abnormality do have an opportunity to describe their experience through the support group publications (SATFA newsletter). This is again a self-selecting group but they describe their experiences very eloquently. There are common themes: a need to share their experience, recalling in precise detail the manner in which they were told that something was wrong, and the personal process by which they came to believe that it was true. They describe their motivations for deciding on termination and their grief experience afterwards. It is clear that a great many women survive intense grief reactions after their terminations and continue to feel very strong emotions triggered by certain events for many years afterwards.

It is as if, for many parents, there is a compulsion to tell because at the time the experience is so personal and remains very isolating, and there are not many people who are able to hear, let alone understand, the detail of what parents go through at this time. Many writers acknowledge that they are sharing their experience as much for themselves as for others who might benefit from reading it. The many 'letters' addressed to unborn children also demonstrate the need to explain and in particular to express the love that motivated the decision. There is no evidence from parents who do not experience the termination as a loss.

Drawing on women's accounts the following dimensions of the experience can be recognised: the stage of the pregnancy, the diagnosis, absorbing information about the baby's condition, the procedure, handling the baby, physical and psychological reactions and the prognosis for future pregnancies.

Psychological impact of termination for fetal abnormality

Much less attention has been paid to the psychological impact of termination for fetal abnormality compared with early termination of pregnancy for other reasons (Blumberg 1984). While the incidence is lower this is possibly because it is seen as a less controversial non-choice. The research that has been done confirms the normality of a grief reaction. In a study of 48 women (Lloyd and Laurence 1985) a grief reaction likened to that following stillbirth was reported by three-quarters of the sample, with nearly a half experiencing symptoms after six months. An additional feature of grief after a termination for abnormality is the burden of responsibility of having made the decision to end the pregnancy. Whilst it is quite common for parents to question the decision they have made the majority of women resolve their ambivalence satisfactorily (White-van Mourik *et al.* 1992).

Although most women continue to feel sad about the loss of their baby research indicates that a small but significant proportion of women (around 20 per cent) continue to feel angry, guilty, a failure, irritable and tearful two years after the termination (White-van Mourik *et al.* 1992). An indicator of difficult adjustment would seem to be ambivalence about the decision, which is likely to be present with non-lethal abnormalities (Shusterman 1979). Gestation at the time of the termination is not thought to be significant but maternal age is – the younger, the harder it is to withstand it – as are previous stressful life-events (Zeanah *et al.* 1993). It has been suggested that non-invasive diagnostic techniques are harder to come to terms with

(White-van Mourik *et al.* 1992), possibly because there is less advance consideration by the woman of the diagnostic component of the tests.

❏ Issues in health care

Whilst it is recognised, from a woman's point of view, that the management of the termination is a significant part of the experience, evaluation of care has not kept pace with changes in practice. The significance of recent changes in the management of early termination, in particular the impact of day surgery, is not clear. Research has focused on identifying problems and little is known of the majority of women for whom there is no identified clinical aftermath.

As with stillbirth and miscarriage health care is a prominent feature of women's reports of their experiences of termination for abnormality. The management of the diagnosis, preparation for labour, information about the abnormality, the attitudes of staff and the frequent lack of routine follow-up care all feature in women's accounts of their experiences. The studies that have been carried out reflect these concerns and refer to the damage caused by insensitive care at the time (for example White-van Mourik *et al.* 1990). Earlier studies identify the poor handling of the baby and the lack of mementoes (Leschot *et al.* 1982) as particular problems. There is reason to believe that women may have benefited in the interim from changes in practice introduced following stillbirth. SATFA has done much to address these issues in terms of the publications for parents and professionals (SATFA 1995) and work with health professionals.

❏ The impact on health professionals

Doctors, nurses and midwives do not have to be involved with the termination of pregnancy. The incidence of conscientious objection is not known, as refusal does not have to be public. Some say nurses cannot work on gynaecological wards if they are not prepared to care for these women (Hulme 1983). There is little discussion of the issues in professional journals.

Although there is increasing awareness of the need to prepare and support staff well, mainly from those concerned with identifying high standards of care, the professional reaction to the termination of pregnancy is not well documented. There is little discussion of the personal resources needed. Although good care demands skilled staff, it is not known how best to acquire these skills. There is little evaluation of the stress that the work places on staff or the most effective ways in which they can deal with it. There is also a wider team of professionals who come into contact with termination, particularly anaesthetists and theatre staff; little is known about the effect on them.

■ The SANDS *Guidelines*

❏ A reflection of changing attitudes

Changes in attitudes to pregnancy loss are both reflected in and promoted by the SANDS *Guidelines,* which address issues of providing a high standard of care. There have been three editions of the *Guidelines* spanning nine years (1986–95), which reflect a gradual developmental process. At each stage something new has been included whilst decisions have also been made to exclude other aspects of pregnancy loss.

The *Guidelines* were first published in 1986 and were confined to stillbirth and neonatal death. Although there were concerns about the care of women who miscarried in the second trimester and a recognition of the arbitrary nature of the gestational divide between miscarriage and stillbirth (then at 28 weeks gestation) a pragmatic decision was taken to keep within the legal boundaries of stillbirth and neonatal death.

The second edition in 1991 included miscarriage along with stillbirth and neonatal death. The division between stillbirth and miscarriage (reduced from 28 to 24 weeks gestation in October 1992) was challenged. There is the implicit assumption that pregnancy loss can be viewed as a continuum of experience, that early loss is not the same as a stillbirth but is nevertheless something that matters. Thinking in terms of the principles behind good practice rather than purely the specifics of what should and should not be done helped identify the common issues. Recognition is given to the uniqueness of experience and the importance of understanding individual needs.

The third edition of the *Guidelines* was published in 1995, and included the termination of pregnancy for any reason, an indication of how much opinions had changed in the intervening four years. In the preface Nancy Kohner wrote:

> There is now a readier understanding among both professionals and
> bereaved families that no matter when or how a pregnancy ends or a
> baby dies, there are some common elements in parents' experience of
> loss and some common needs. Most important for professional carers,
> there are principles of good practice that are relevant for every kind of
> loss.   (SANDS 1995 p4)

Including voluntary pregnancy loss in this way, acknowledging that there were similarities as well as differences between a termination for abnormality and late miscarriage or stillbirth or that there could be aspects of loss to the early termination of pregnancy was a radical new departure.

The *Guidelines* have been widely publicised and largely welcomed by the health professionals at whom they are aimed. The endorsement of the second edition by the *House of Commons Health Committee Inquiry into Maternity Services* (HMSO 1992a) and the government response (Maternity

Services, HMSO 1992b), recommending the implementation of the *Guidelines* and the appropriate training of staff, were clear indications of the concern about provision in this area.

❑ Development of the SANDS *Guidelines*

The *Guidelines* came about in response to the concern and anger expressed by parents at the way in which stillbirth and neonatal death were managed in hospital. SANDS was also aware of the disparity in professional practice throughout the country. It had also become clear that some professionals were uneasy in the role the current system of care imposed upon them. There were sympathetic professionals whose concerns reflected parents' views and who were receptive to the improvements in care that were needed.

There was a consensus within SANDS that the best way forward was to identify both the professionals responsible and the places where good practice existed. The recommendations in the *Guidelines* specify the nature of good care and draw on examples of good practice in particular localities. The focus is not on poor care, which was defined only by implication. Extensive research was undertaken into areas of good practice in consultation with interested parties, both lay and professional. This is the basis of the *Guidelines*; they are not based on systematic research of specific aspects of care reviewed over a period of time.

The process of the development of the *Guidelines* was crucial. A working party was set up composed of representatives at a senior level of all the major professional bodies as well as the voluntary organisations. The working party debated many complex issues, including the relevance of gestation, the comparisons between voluntary and involuntary loss, the complexities, both emotional and practical, of sensitive disposal arrangements and the appropriateness of the term 'baby', as well as considering the specific recommendations that should be made.

So the recommendations are based on the views of both parents/women (albeit arguably a biased group who contact self-help organisations) and of professionals. In contrast to much of the rhetoric about patient-led care the development of the *Guidelines* is a very good example of how consumers of services have initiated change, but in conjunction with professionals who have been sensitive to their needs. There has been genuine co-operation between the users of services and professionals based on a recognition of the expertise both bring to the dilemmas that are faced.

The *Guidelines* represent a shift in view of what is considered good practice. Twenty-five years ago professional practice aimed to protect women from their experience. Broadly speaking, today the task of the health professional in consultation with the woman is to help her to face up to the reality of her experience. This clearly imposes far-reaching demands on both women as patients and the professionals who care for them. A strength of the *Guidelines* is that the implications for professionals are acknowledged. Greater understanding by service users about professional needs is promoted. It is recognised that providing the sort of care recommended is demanding and difficult work. Health professionals need support and training to do it.

❏ Limitations of the *Guidelines*

It is important to view these developments as a beginning. At best, guidelines focus on important issues and are an impetus to develop policy and improve practice. At worst, they become a list of things to be ticked off, giving the illusion that needs are being met and effective help given. The very fact of their existence can distance practitioners from the reality of the experience they need to understand. To be of any use at all guidelines have to be read and put into practice. Their effectiveness will depend on the skill of practitioners to understand and implement them.

Without appropriate training and management support guidelines will have little impact on services. Moreover, there are gaps in our knowledge and limited material available on which to base training and advise health practitioners. The National Extension College Training Pack (Kohner and Leftwich 1995) provides a basis for training staff. Experiential learning methods are used to help staff to understand their own and others' reactions to emotionally demanding and distressing situations and to develop their skills in dealing with them. However, the broader issues concerning the implications of providing these qualities of care in this area have not been addressed.

■ The study

The intention of this book is to begin to redress the balance. The research, funded by the Department of Health, was designed to underpin the SANDS *Guidelines* and to address the issues for both women and health professionals. The study focuses on the interface between patient and professional in the context of a local health care system and gives insight into the complexities of providing the care that is currently advocated. The reader can enter the worlds of all the participants as well as considering more objectively the strategies for equipping staff to do the job and improving professional practice. It is hoped that, in placing their own experience against that described in the study, readers will be able to make greater sense of the strengths and weaknesses of the system of care of which they are a part.

The overall purpose of the project was to increase understanding of women's experiences of pregnancy loss with a view to assisting health professionals to improve their professional practice. Stillbirth, miscarriage and termination of pregnancy (for whatever reason) were included. It therefore reflected the contemporary view implicit in the SANDS *Guidelines* that pregnancy loss can be viewed as a continuum of experience. The research was a case study of the experience and management of pregnancy loss in one hospital which serves a largely urban population of about 200,000 in southern England.

A qualitative approach was adopted. The study consisted of semi-structured, in-depth interviews with 20 women selected to represent the different categories of pregnancy loss, together with the 70 health professionals (obstetricians, gynaecologists, anaesthetists, nurses, midwives, sonographers, GPs and a health visitor) whom they identified as being significant in their care. Funding did not allow for the women's partners to be included. Detailed information was gained about the system of care in the hospital in order to put the women's and health professionals' experiences into context. Appendix I explains the methods adopted for the study in more detail.

The study provides a snapshot of women's and health professionals' experiences at one particular point in time. Ideally, the study should be replicated in other areas. However, even though this hospital was unique in its history and character, as were the women and health professionals, it was in many other respects probably not dissimilar to many in the country. Although the precise nature of the strengths and weaknesses in care will vary between hospitals and with individuals the principles that underpin that care are likely to be similar and there will therefore be lessons to be learned from the in-depth study in one location.

Chapters 2, 3 and 4 consider women's and health professionals' perspectives on health care. The book has been organised according to the categories of experience (early miscarriage, early termination and second- and third-trimester loss) in order to make the material easily accessible to a wide range of readers. Each chapter outlines the system of care and background information about the women before considering aspects of health care in more detail, incorporating both women's and health professionals' views. Chapter 5 considers the personal impact of the work on the health professionals. Chapter 6 draws together the implications of the study.

■ Suggestions for further reading

A full bibliography of texts which have informed the study are listed at the end of the book. At the end of each of the following chapters suggestions are made for further reading. These are intended to amplify points made in the text and help the reader to take further some of the issues raised in the text. It is not an exhaustive list.

General texts which the practitioner working in this area may find useful are listed below.

Kohner, N. and Leftwich, A. (1995) *Pregnancy Loss and the Death of a Baby. A Training Pack*, Cambridge, National Extension College.
Mander, R. (1994) *Loss and Bereavement in Childbearing*, Oxford, Blackwell Scientific.
SANDS (1995) *Pregnancy Loss and the Death of a Baby: Guidelines for Professionals*, London, SANDS.
Schott, J. and Henley, A. (1996) *Culture, Religion and Childbearing in a Multiracial Society*, Oxford, Butterworth-Heinemann.
Stewart, A. and Dent, A. (1994) *At a Loss: Bereavement Care When a Baby Dies*, Eastbourne, Baillière Tindall.

Chapter 2

Early miscarriage

■ **Introduction**

❏ **The local health care system**

Women in early pregnancy who experience the symptoms of miscarriage, (spotting, bleeding, cramps and no longer feeling pregnant) normally consult their GP. Some women may be unaware of problems with their pregnancy, which are only discovered during a routine consultation with their GP or midwife or at a routine ultrasound scan. In this locality the GP will refer the woman to the local hospital where she will be seen in the Early Pregnancy Assessment Clinic (EPAC) in the Accident and Emergency (A&E) department by a gynaecology SHO who will examine her, organise an ultrasound scan and, if necessary, arrange admission to the emergency ward for an ERPC. At the time of this study, in this hospital, it was routine practice that miscarrying women be admitted for an ERPC. The medical management of miscarriage was not available and it was very unusual for a woman diagnosed as miscarrying not to have an ERPC.

Routine follow-up of miscarriage patients is not undertaken: women are advised to see their GP. Since the recruitment of the women to the study the role of the bereavement counsellor on the maternity unit has been extended to include women on the emergency ward. This service was not available to women at the time of this study

The current system of health care is characterised by the lack of contact between health professional and patient. The stay in hospital is brief and movement through the system rapid, from A&E via the ultrasound department to the emergency ward and including a trip to theatre often within 24 hours, each department forming a link in the chain of care. Contact and communication between the different departments and professionals is often limited. As a consequence it is common for health professionals to lack knowledge about the care available to women before and after they see her. It is a system that is described by health professionals as 'being processed' and by the women as 'passing from pillar to post', a system in which it is easy to ignore the psychological aspects of care.

❏ The women

Background information

Table 2.1   Early miscarriage: background information

	Age	Relationship with partner	Occupation
Pauline	32	cohab/stable relationship	stewardess
Laura	29	cohab/unstable relationship	part-time waitress
Katy	18	married	housewife/mother (never worked)
Carol	24	single short-term relationship	unemployed
Val	25	cohab/stable relationship	hairdresser
Ann	33	married	housewife (clerical worker)

Table 2.1 summarises the background information about the women. They ranged in age from 18 to 33 years. All of the women described their partner as being supportive at the time of the miscarriage although the nature of their relationships differed. Four of the women considered their relationship with their partner stable and long term; Katy and Ann were married, Val and Pauline both cohabiting. Laura and Carol considered their relationship with their partners to be unstable and short term but described their partners as involved and supportive throughout the miscarriage, accompanying them to hospital and caring for them afterwards.

The women differed in their experience of pregnancy (Table 2.2). Apart from Pauline, who was pregnant for the first time, the others had all been pregnant before. Only Katy had a child. Laura, Carol and Val had, at some point in the past, had a termination of pregnancy. None of them had regrets about the termination but, when discussing their current miscarriage, all made frequent reference to the termination and compared the experiences.

Table 2.2   Early miscarriage: women's experiences of pregnancy

	Reproductive history	Women's views about this pregnancy
Pauline	first pregnancy	planned and wanted but sooner than expected
Laura	TOP age 18	not using contraception but unplanned; had decided on termination
Katy	preterm delivery of daughter now $2^1/2$; miscarriage at 20 weeks	planned and wanted
Carol	TOP 12 months ago	an 'accident'; considered termination but decided against it
Val	TOP age 18	planned and wanted but earlier than expected
Ann	two ectopic pregnancies seven years' infertility	'longed for'; first of two chances at IVF

TOP = termination of pregnancy.

Katy and Ann had a history of reproductive problems. Following the premature birth of her daughter and a miscarriage at 20 weeks gestation Katy had been diagnosed as having an incompetent cervix. As a consequence this pregnancy was carefully monitored and, had the pregnancy continued, a 'stitch' (Shirodkar suture) would have been inserted. Ann had a history of infertility. She had been trying for a baby for seven years and, as a result of two ectopic pregnancies, had become unable to conceive. The pregnancy she miscarried was the result of IVF, the first of her two chances funded by the NHS.

Women's experiences of this pregnancy

Apart from Laura and Carol all the women had planned, if not longed, to be pregnant, even if it had happened sooner than they had expected. Their feelings ranged from surprise to pleasure and excitement. In addition Katy and Ann, who because of their reproductive difficulties valued their pregnancies highly, were also fearful that it would go wrong again.

Laura's pregnancy was unplanned although she had not been using contraception and had, according to her GP, decided to terminate the pregnancy. She miscarried before the outpatient appointment to arrange a termination was booked. In contrast Carol had become pregnant accidentally and seriously considered a termination, seeking a consultation with her GP to discuss this, but had decided to continue with the pregnancy. She felt she had made a very conscious decision to 'keep the baby' and had become very involved in the pregnancy.

Table 2.3 contrasts the ideas the women had about their pregnancies with their knowledge of the physical reality of the miscarriage. Early pregnancy is recognised as a time of ambivalence and uncertainty, of forming an attachment to the baby and of facing up to the reality of the pregnancy and of a baby in some months' time. It is clear that these women were at different stages along this road, as indicated by changes in their behaviour and the courses of action they had taken. They had told people about the pregnancy, bought or collected things for the baby and given the baby a name or nickname. For all of them the baby clearly had an emotional reality. The understanding they had developed contrasted with the physical reality of the baby at the time of the miscarriage.

Women's experiences of the miscarriage

Table 2.4 summarises the women's experiences of the miscarriage. For three of the women the miscarriage was physically or medically dramatic. They all miscarried later in their pregnancy (12–14 weeks). Laura bled very heavily and was in pain; she was admitted to hospital at night as a medical emergency. Carol, who had not recognised the spotting as symptoms

Table 2.3 Early miscarriage: women's ideas about the pregnancy compared with the physical reality of the miscarriage

	Women's ideas about the pregnancy/baby	Women's knowledge of the physical reality	Women's unasked questions
Pauline	thinking about preparing the baby's room; her mother had bought things for the baby; had told family and friends but not colleagues	at scan 'nothing there'	
Laura	thought what the baby would look like; had told friends; thought how she would be as a mother	heavy bleeding, large clot removed by SHO in A&E (NB: SHO removed complete sac with embryo)	was the clot the baby?
Katy	told family and friends; 'took things slower', looked after herself; rest and good food; had begun to think of names	at scan 'nothing there'	what was removed at the ERPC?
Carol	had told friends and family; played music to the baby; gave the baby a nickname	at scan saw small fetus; passed large clot after scan but didn't want to look	was the clot the baby?
Val	had not told family but told friends at work; had a name for the baby; thought about decorating the spare room; bought the baby a teddy	at scan 'womb empty'; bleeding prior to scan included large clot	was the clot the baby?
Ann	'they were babies to me' (reference to current miscarriage and ectopic pregnancies); due to reproductive history and anxiety about success of pregnancy thought in medical terms of developing embryo	scan showed pregnancy not viable	what was removed at ERPC?

of a threatened miscarriage, also experienced heavy bleeding and pain and became very anxious. Pauline, who said her miscarriage had been described to her as a 'textbook blighted ovum', was apparently a more straightforward case. She had experienced slight spotting but thought this was normal. However, it was feared that, during the ERPC, her womb had been punctured (although it had not) and a laparoscopy was necessary.

Table 2.4 Early miscarriage: the miscarriage

	Gestation	Description of miscarriage	Women's realisation of the miscarriage	Significance of the miscarriage: women's views
Pauline	14	'textbook blighted ovum'; stopped feeling pregnant five weeks previously; slight spotting	at scan (expected it to be OK)	a hitch on the route to successful pregnancy
Laura	12	very heavy bleeding; emergency admission to hospital; complete sac passed in A&E	when bleeding and cramps became severe	a relief; a trauma; aroused feelings about previous termination and ideals of motherhood
Katy	11	blighted ovum; spotting from very early on	thought it wouldn't work when bleeding started but hopeful until third scan	a medical mishap; aroused memories of previous miscarriage; threatened sense of hope.
Carol	14	missed abortion, scan confirmed baby died three weeks earlier; spotting followed by pain, cramps and heavy loss	at scan (expected it to be OK, ignored SHO and GP)	a turning point in her life; 'grown up'
Val	8	spotting and cramps followed by bleeding and loss of large clots	at scan	aroused feelings about her family rivalry with her sisters; not getting what she wants
Ann	8	bleeding, stopped feeling pregnant very early on	at first scan thought it wouldn't work out; remained optimistic until second scan	intense sense of loss of this and previous babies; loss of hope

In contrast Katy, Val and Ann described their miscarriage as physically inconsequential: light spotting and not feeling pregnant any more. They miscarried earlier in their pregnancy, at 8–12 weeks, but had experienced symptoms drawn out over several days or weeks and had time to recognise that things were going wrong. They described their pregnancies as 'iffy'.

For these six women the experience of their pregnancy and miscarriage was very different. In addition to the contrast in the physical experience of the miscarriage their reactions varied both at the time and later. Each brought with them to the miscarriage a complex web of their personal history, characteristics and expectations as well as their present circumstances and future aspirations, which affected the way they felt about their miscarriage.

Pauline was very straightforward about the miscarriage and, although upset, was optimistic about the future. For her the miscarriage was 'a hitch en route to a successful pregnancy'. Although distressed by the physical trauma Laura was overwhelmingly relieved she had miscarried but troubled by memories of her earlier termination and her ambivalence and ideals of motherhood, which she felt she would never be able to meet. Val was confronted with the rivalry she felt with her sisters and felt isolated and unsupported by her family, who were unaware of her pregnancy. Katy dismissed this miscarriage as 'an insignificant non-event' but her sense of hope was threatened as she relived the loss of her previous pregnancy. Similarly, Ann relived her previous ectopic pregnancies. Her sense of loss of this pregnancy and of hope of a future successful pregnancy was intense.

Their feelings about the miscarriage cannot be neatly linked to the gestation of the pregnancy, their feelings about it nor the physical process of the miscarriage. The emotional reality often bears little relationship to the physical reality but is a result of more hidden feelings of which the woman may herself have been previously unaware and which may surface at the crisis of the miscarriage or afterwards.

❏ Women's experiences of miscarriage: professionals' views

Professionals' attitudes to miscarriage

Most staff when interviewed demonstrated a clear understanding in principle of the significance that a miscarriage may have for a woman and how women's needs may not be met by the current system of care. They recognised the discrepancy between the potential significance of a miscarriage for the individual, for whom it may or may not be a major crisis, and the significance of miscarriage within the health care system, where it is inevitably a routine minor medical event:

> We might see three or four women miscarrying a day and it's very easy from our point of view to think they're two a penny... You know for each individual it's quite a major and traumatic life event to them. There's a lot more to it but I think you are aware of that but you are not really involved in that side. SHO

The hospital-based professionals, in contrast to the GPs, some of whom were involved in the longer term, were dealing with the women at the point of crisis of the miscarriage and recognised that they often did not and could not know how the women felt about it. For some, like the SHO quoted above, it was not part of their job.

Although there was a general understanding that later loss was worse and warranted more recognition it was clear that few professionals took the view that miscarriage did not matter. The importance and consequences of early loss were recognised. As one consultant put it, 'no matter when the baby is lost you've lost the bit in nine months time'. A couple of nurses stressed the deep sense of loss women felt after a miscarriage, saying, 'the gestation of the pregnancy doesn't make much difference' and 'miscarriage is always traumatic but it may take time for feelings to surface'. One GP took the view that miscarriage is 'always a crisis and normally a loss'.

It was also recognised that miscarriage is a diverse experience, which has a unique meaning for the individual and that women react differently to apparently similar events. A nurse describes her understanding of the range of individual experience:

> It depends on the couple I think. Because I mean for somebody who has tried to get pregnant for ten years a baby at eight to ten weeks, it's a nightmare for them to lose that baby. Whereas somebody who has already got three children and perhaps they thought about having a fourth but you know they've had a miscarriage... or they've had to have a termination at 12 weeks... It might be as momentous to them as someone who has been trying to get pregnant for ten years but it might not. But I think it's so individual. Some people from the time they are pregnant would feel devastated if they lost the baby, other people don't think of babies as babies until they start feeling them moving around.

Understanding the complexity of early miscarriage

Although the understanding of miscarriage in general terms was good, professionals' thinking about the complexity of early pregnancy and the different ways women interpret this was much more muddled. Asking someone to define when they think a baby is a baby rather than a pregnancy or a bunch of cells or something that will be something in the future is a complex task, drawing on their personal and professional experiences and personal belief system. An understanding of this issue is, however, fundamental in understanding how professionals respond to women who miscarry. Clearly, some individuals will be more sophisticated in their response, more reflective and articulate, and comfortable in thinking in abstract concepts, whilst others will be more concrete and pragmatic.

Attitudes and understanding of the experience of miscarriage develop over time. It was common for those interviewed to refer to a particular personal experience of pregnancy or that of a friend, or to their professional experience, as instrumental in developing their understanding. For example, a student nurse talked eloquently of the personal consequences of a termination of pregnancy and how that had changed her views. An SHO described her surprise at her friend's devastation after a miscarriage. A registrar talked of the experience of his wife's pregnancy and the birth of his children. A GP had been profoundly influenced in her ideas by her professional experience working as an anaesthetist for an abortion clinic.

A few health professionals found the question difficult to answer, either because they had not thought about it (SHO) or because it was too difficult to think about (registrar). One consultant, although willing and able to discuss the issue at length, said he preferred not to think about it like that:

I must admit – I don't think about it in those terms usually. I mean because it would be very difficult if you spent... a lot of the work would become very incredibly difficult to square with yourself if you spent hours talking about when is a baby? When is it not a baby? When is it a gamete? When is it a fetus? And all this – it isn't particularly helpful. It isn't particularly helpful.

The health professionals interviewed for this study had a range of views, as the following quotes illustrate:

It's a very individual thing. I mean I define a baby as a baby from conception. And that's based on my religious beliefs perhaps but also based on the fact that I knew when I was pregnant from the first weeks, you know I began to relate to a being within myself so that's a very individual thing. That's not an opinion that I could say was everybody's.   GP

Ah... it's a baby... once they see an image... I think prior to that it probably varies from woman to woman doesn't it? She has a scan at six weeks, it's a bit of a sac. She has a scan at eight weeks, may be there's a bit more. A missed abortion at ten weeks, it's an amorphous blob. So I don't know if it's right actually.   Registrar obstetrician

I think I would define a baby from an ordinary woman's point of view from the moment of conception really because even if you... I mean I lost a baby at 12 weeks, but it was still my baby. And I know it wasn't a baby in the true sense of the word but it was still my baby and I still lost it and we still grieve. So I think that immediately a lady knows that she is pregnant and then she loses her baby, it's a baby. I don't think women call it a fetus.   Midwife

I think it's a baby from the beginning... I think it's traumatic... it's always a baby but the further into the gestation it goes, the worse it can get because the baby is obvious... you've been carrying it for longer as well so the people have actually bonded with it for a longer period of time.   Emergency ward nurse

To me I think a baby is a baby when it is born, you know, alive and healthy.   Staff nurse, emergency ward

I think the legal definition of 24 weeks is the most reasonable.
                                                                  Registrar anaesthetist

One tends to look at it from the point of view of what attachment and ties that the mother or the pregnant woman has. And if they've made a connection then it's a real entity to them.   Registrar obstetrician

I don't have any problems with it actually because I think of these early pregnancies as not even a live pregnancy which is why I don't personally have any problems with terminations. I don't find any difficulty with that.   SHO

For some women once she knows she's pregnant – depends on how wanted this pregnancy is and how philosophical you can be about a malformed, blighted ovum.   GP

I guess it becomes a baby when you decide... perhaps when you decide you want to go ahead for the pregnancy, that honestly is the best definition I think. It's a baby from the time two cells unite, but no, it becomes a baby from the moment you decide to call it your baby.
          Registrar anaesthetist

When the woman feels the baby move.   Health visitor

From 12 weeks onwards because it's recognisable at that stage.   SHO

Once the pregnancy is confirmed.   Nurse

It is clear from this range of definitions that different criteria were used as a basis for the definition varying from the biological – it's a baby from conception – to a more rigid but arbitrary definition based on gestation: nine weeks, 10–12 weeks viability or birth. The professionals opting for definitions at a later stage acknowledged that, for them, this view 'makes it much easier emotionally', that early termination and early miscarriage were not problematic to them because they were not to do with the loss of a baby.

Others linked the idea of a baby to the characteristics of the baby or to the mother's knowledge or perception of certain characteristics, to when the baby becomes tangible and can be seen on the screen, when the fetal heart can be heard or the woman can feel the baby move. This type of definition is particularly difficult when women miscarry. Several nurses thought that women's understanding that there was a baby and their reactions to it were linked to the actual presence of a fetus and that women were more upset if they saw it, the implication being that if there were no fetus or if women did not see it they would not think in terms of the loss of a baby and would not be so upset. As the understanding that a woman has of the emotional reality of the pregnancy and the physical reality are not necessarily the same this inaccurate grasp of the complexity of miscarriage has profound implications for the quality of understanding that these health professionals are able to offer their patients.

The most striking difference in the definitions given was in the focus given to the women's experience, whether the importance of the women's definition of the pregnancy was stressed or the health professionals imposed their own view. Since women's definitions vary there is clearly a risk in getting it wrong if rigid criteria are employed. Sticking with a woman's definition, whatever that may be, also means accepting any conflict there may be with the professional's personal views.

In contrast to the doctors and nurses, for whom there was no clear pattern of reactions, the midwives interviewed demonstrated a clear woman-centred understanding of the complexity and potential significance of early loss. Perhaps their detailed knowledge of pregnancy and their involvement in antenatal care and the care of women who may have miscarried in a previous pregnancy provides them with ample evidence of the nature and consequences of miscarriage; midwives are not normally involved in caring for women who miscarry.

❏ Overall evaluation of health care

Women's views

All the women felt well cared for medically, describing their medical care as prompt and efficient. On the whole the women described the hospital staff as kind, friendly and helpful. Many examples were given of when understanding and sensitive care were particularly appreciated, often in exchanges that only took a few minutes but were nevertheless important: the anaesthetist who was reassuring and understood one woman's fear of anaesthetics; the SHO who understood another's irrational fear of a hysterectomy; the nurse who competently and caringly dealt with heavy bleeding after the ERPC; the registrar who calmed a woman's panic about the ERPC; and the porter who made one woman who was feeling very neglected laugh. Only two unhelpful comments were reported by the women. One woman described the duty GP as very brusque when he informed her that she had miscarried and another was upset that when her partner asked the SHO if she could drink wine the evening she got home he suggested that they were going to celebrate.

However, the women differed in their views of their overall health care. Table 2.5 summarises the women's perceptions of different aspects of their care. Qualitative differences in the care the women received as well as their different characteristics and expectations contributed to their views.

Pauline, Laura and Carol defined their health care as good:

It was fine.

I was quite impressed. I didn't come away feeling that was terrible, it was only the pain that was terrible.

It was good. I couldn't identify any improvements. Excellent.

Table 2.5   Early miscarriage: women's perceptions of care

	GP care		Assessment in A&E/EPAC	Ultrasound care	Inpatient care	Management of discharge from hospital
	Before admission to hospital	After admission to hospital				
Pauline	1	1	1	2	2	5
Laura	2	–	1	–	1	3
Katy	2	5	4	1	5	5
Carol	1	1	1	1	1	4
Val	3	5	5/1	2	5	4
Ann	5	5	–	–	5	5

1 = very helpful
2 = helpful
3 = neither helpful nor unhelpful
4 = unhelpful
5 = very unhelpful
– = no experience of this aspect of care

They clearly felt their needs were met and were appreciative of the help they were given. These women all felt they had a GP they could trust; they had a sense of a competent doctor on their side. They had the support of their partners throughout their hospital stay and were cared for at a time when the hospital was less busy than usual. Pauline and Carol also had the opportunity to prepare for their hospital admission.

These women were medically or emotionally demanding. Laura's miscarriage was a medical emergency and Carol became very agitated before the miscarriage and bled heavily after the ERPC. It was feared that Pauline's womb had been punctured during the ERPC. For these women the staff had an obvious medical role to play and the women thought they did it well and felt safe. In addition none of these women, during their hospital admission, wanted to talk about their feelings either because they felt too ill and wanted to sleep or because they wanted to maintain a 'chatty' relationship with the staff 'to keep their mind off things'. They did not want anyone to probe.

In contrast Katy, Val and Ann defined their care as poor:

It was quite awful actually.

It was awful especially when you've got no-one with you. It was only a minor thing so they left me.

They felt alone, abandoned, ignored and unknown. They said no-one really talked to them, which they explained in terms of miscarriage being 'unimportant', 'other people being really ill' and 'the staff were very nice but they were so busy'. These women were not obviously ill or needy. They were not medically difficult or demanding in terms of this miscarriage and were probably quiet and conforming in hospital.

They all experienced delays or long waits in their care and all of them said they had hardly spoken to anybody whilst they were in hospital. For a while they had recognised that things might be or were going wrong with their pregnancy and had been getting, or trying to get, medical help. None of them felt they had a GP whom they could really trust and all three women were on their own for much of the time they were in hospital. Although all had long-term, stable relationships their partners were not actively supportive to them whilst they were in hospital. They were hard to contact, had other very young children to look after, were so upset themselves or could not stand hospitals.

In different ways these women were anomalies in the system, which was not prepared for them. The inattentiveness of her GP meant that Val referred herself to the A&E department and was not booked in to the EPAC. She was inexperienced in terms of pregnancy and hospital care and was overwhelmed by the institution. Ann missed EPAC and was booked straight in to the emergency ward from the private hospital, with which she compared her care unfavourably. Katy had been in and out of EPAC and was an 'old hand'. For Katy and Ann their reproductive problems meant there was a history to this particular miscarriage as well as, in their view, previous experiences of poor care and negative events in this hospital.

Health professionals' views

As with the women a high standard of medical care was taken for granted by the health professionals but criticism of the system of care for women who miscarry was common, particularly from doctors. The GPs were concerned about the service the hospital provided, about women getting lost in an 'unsympathetic system' and about the time it takes to get a scan organised, although it was recognised that the EPAC should improve this. The SHOs and registrars were critical of the system in which they had to work:

> ERPCs get very bad treatment; they are low priority, frequent and routine. From our point of view they are an irritation which probably comes across... they get bumped down the emergency list, they are largely ignored.   Registrar

> I think our care and support of those, the early ones, is cruel... Maybe because of the numbers... you just haven't got the time to give them the support... I think perhaps we should.   Registrar

> For her medical needs I think it was fine. She came in and she had it done in the afternoon... and she went home presumably bleeding... And from a medical point of view I am sure it was fine. And it does run smoothly when it runs like that. But I don't think that having lost a baby that you really wanted and being able to talk about it or grieve, no I don't think we handled that... well I didn't approach it at

all. I don't know if the nurse did. But I don't think basically we do
well on that aspect.   SHO

For health professionals, anxious to provide a good service for women
which meets their needs, working within a system that makes it difficult to
do that can be undermining and a source of tension. The doctors were
surprised that women were as positive as they were about their health care.

■ Health care prior to admission to hospital

❏ GP care prior to admission to hospital

The amount and nature of the contact the women had with their GP prior to
their hospital admission varied (Table 2.6). The GPs described their initial
task with women consulting them with problems in early pregnancy as accurate assessment and organising appropriate referral. In this pregnancy Ann
had no contact with her GP as she was undergoing infertility treatment at
another hospital and her GP was not involved. The women's feelings about
the pregnancy influenced the initial approach they made to their GPs. Laura
and Carol initially consulted their GPs to discuss termination of pregnancy
whereas Katy, because of problems in previous pregnancies, regularly saw
her doctor for antenatal care from early on.

Apart from Ann all the women consulted their GP with symptoms of
bleeding and concerns about the pregnancy. Only Katy, who was booked for
consultant care, was referred directly to the hospital for a scan for an assessment of the viability of the pregnancy. Val was falsely reassured and twice
told, by different doctors, to go away and come back if the bleeding
increased. The bleeding did not get worse but persisted and, on the advice of
a colleague, she referred herself to the A&E department. Laura phoned the
GP and described her symptoms. She was advised to seek help if the
bleeding worsened but an appointment was made for her to see the GP in a
week's time to discuss her request for a termination. Both women felt their
symptoms were not taken seriously by the GP and felt 'fobbed off'.

Pauline and Carol were both initially seen by a locum or a duty GP
who reassured them about their symptoms. The next day their own GP,
concerned about their symptoms, referred them to the EPAC at the hospital
(see below). In both cases the GP, believing women have a right to know
whether a pregnancy is viable as soon as possible and anxious for the
woman's welfare owing to the severity of the symptoms reported, was
critical that the first doctor had not made the referral immediately. A lack
of knowledge about the local service arrangements may have contributed
to this.

For the women the route to hospital was rarely straightforward.
However, only Val was overtly critical of her GP practice. Pauline, Laura,
Katy and Carol all had a GP at the practice where they were registered

Table 2.6 Early miscarriage: GP care prior to hospital admission (this pregnancy)

	Woman has a GP she identifies as 'her doctor'	Contact with GP	Women's views	GP's views
Pauline	✓	locum GP reassured her when consulted about spotting; telephone call from own GP (who had checked the locum's work) telling her to go to EPAC the next day for a scan; telephone call from GP to discuss scan result	GP understanding and helpful	alarmed that locum had not referred her for a scan
Laura	✓	initial consultation to confirm pregnancy and discuss termination; awaiting appointment with second GP to arrange termination as first GP unwilling to do so; telephone call to first GP to discuss bleeding; advised to wait for appointment with second GP in several days time; emergency GP called out at night due to heavy bleeding; referred straight to hospital	thought bleeding not taken seriously enough by first GP because of decision to terminate pregnancy; duty GP brusque in telling her she was miscarrying	first GP gave her a lot of time, information and advice; thought she should have arranged to see her own GP sooner
Katy	✓	antenatal care careful monitoring due to previous problems in pregnancy – early referral to consultant; frequent contact re spotting and scan results	antenatal care good; at the time thought GP understanding and supportive; in retrospect angry that GP was not straight with her after first scan, thought GP conspired with hospital against her	did best possible in the circumstances
Carol	✓	to confirm pregnancy and discuss termination (decided to continue with pregnancy); symptoms of miscarriage, home visit by duty GP, reassured; next day saw own GP, referred to EPAC	when considering termination felt pressurised by GP to continue with pregnancy; when miscarrying felt well cared for	duty GP should have referred her to EPAC
Val	✗	appointment in surgery; GP reassured her re bleeding; 3 days later saw another GP, again reassured re bleeding (NB: she referred herself to A&E on the advice of a friend)	felt 'fobbed off' by GP who ignored her symptoms and was unsympathetic	not interviewed
Ann	✗	no contact (undergoing IVF treatment at another hospital; GP not involved)	—	—

whom they referred to as 'their doctor' even though this doctor was not seen at the first consultation. All these women felt positive about their GP care although Katy later turned against her GP, critical of what she described as the GP's lack of honesty over the probable negative outcome of her pregnancy. She felt that it had been clear from the first scan (she had three) and that nobody had been straight with her – she had been 'strung along'. The professionals involved were merely being cautious and waiting for a clear scan result.

■ Hospital care

❑ Arrival at hospital

A&E department/EPAC

Women referred to this hospital with problems in their pregnancy are seen in the A&E department by the SHO. Their history is taken, they are examined and referred for an ultrasound scan after which they return to A&E for further discussions with the SHO.

Coincidental with the recruitment of participants to this study, an Early Pregnancy Assessment Clinic (EPAC) was set up in the hospital's A&E department. The aim of EPAC is to streamline the service for women with problem pregnancies by reducing the waiting time in A&E and for theatre. The clinic operates for one hour in the morning when the gynaecology SHO is available to see women booked in by their GP. The clinic is staffed by a nursing auxiliary allocated for the morning from the antenatal clinic, who talks to the women and acts as chaperone. An hour is allocated during which women can be seen in the ultrasound department and later in the day an hour of theatre time is set aside for women who need an ERPC. Clearly it takes time to establish such a service and, when the women in this study were interviewed, the clinic was in its infancy.

Staff generally considered that the organisation of the EPAC enabled them to provide a more efficient service, women were less likely to wait a long time and it was easier to organise their care although it was stressed that it did not address women's wider needs. Concern was expressed by several junior doctors that the EPAC was perceived as 'a bit of a nuisance in A&E'. A registrar thought that a trained nurse should be allocated to the clinic.

Apart from Ann, who was admitted straight to the emergency ward following referral from the private hospital where her miscarriage had been confirmed, the women were all admitted through A&E. Laura was admitted as an emergency in the middle of the night, the others through the EPAC. Pauline and Carol were referred by their GP, Katy was sent to the EPAC following the diagnosis of a miscarriage at a repeat scan and Val, having referred herself to A&E, was told to come back the next day to the EPAC.

The women were at different stages in understanding what was happening to them. These differences between the women when they arrived at hospital were in the areas of:

- the extent and duration of the physical symptoms
- the woman's interpretation of her symptoms
- her health care prior to arrival at hospital
- being alone or accompanied by her partner, friend or relative
- the meaning and significance of the pregnancy.

Women's views

They had already taken my details over the phone from my GP and while standing at reception they were asking my boyfriend my date of birth, where I lived, etc. and I was standing there bleeding. You know I was in agony, blood was just pouring from me, I was in my dressing gown. And I just said, 'For God's sake please just, you know, do something'. So they put me in a chair and then put me onto a stretcher and put me in this room, where a gynaecologist came to see me. And from there on after it was all OK. The nurses were very pleasant, everyone explained what was going on and I was then taken to the ward.

Laura

I was in the waiting room about ten minutes and then I went straight through into a cubicle and waited for the nurse to come and ask questions... I mean they ask you about four or five times. And they write it down four or five times. I got up there [hospital] about one o'clock... He did an internal to feel if my cervix was open and he tried doing a smear, just have a look but the light wasn't working so he couldn't do it. And he took some blood and I've got some nice marks there. And I was given a drip because I wasn't allowed to eat or drink anything so I wouldn't get thirsty. And then eventually at about four thirty I went up the ward.

Katy

When I first went I was there about five minutes and then went straight through to see the doctor, then we walked to the scan and waited about ten minutes, took me about that long to drink the jug of water... But when I came back from the scan I had to wait about half an hour, 40 minutes, to see the doctor again. And I was waiting in the main waiting room and I was very upset and there were a couple of drunks there and he'd broke his hand and they did quite a lot of shouting. I was on my own at that stage... After about half an hour I asked the nurse if there was somewhere quiet I could sit.

Carol

Arrival at hospital, anxious about the viability of your pregnancy, possibly in pain, is stressful, as these women described. However smoothly the system works it is unlikely that waiting time can be eliminated. The women who were attending a planned appointment or defined as a medical emergency were all seen promptly by the duty SHO but nevertheless said that 'there was a lot of hanging about'. The A&E department can be a frightening place to be. The waiting areas are very public and, if you are vulnerable, can feel dangerous. The cubicles offer little privacy and the staff are often busy. It is experienced, by staff and women alike, as an unpleasant place to be and it is generally accepted by the staff that it is a far from ideal place for women who are miscarrying. One registrar described it as a 'hell hole' and argued that the service would be significantly improved if it were moved to a more sympathetic location such as a gynaecology ward.

In streamlining the service the EPAC reduces the 'hanging about time' in hospital and, unless it is an emergency, enables a woman's admission to hospital to be planned. Pauline and Carol were booked in for an ERPC the following day. They had time to go home and prepare themselves for an admission to hospital. Katy and Val, in contrast, do not appear to have been given this option and were admitted to the hospital for an ERPC later the same day. As a consequence both women experienced long waits in the A&E department after the ultrasound scan before they could be admitted to the ward. They were on their own and had no opportunity to go home or to prepare themselves. If this situation could have been avoided they may not have felt so negative about their hospital care.

❏ The ultrasound scan

The ultrasound department

The ultrasound department is some way from the A&E department, in cramped unsatisfactory conditions in the basement of a different building; at the time of this study renovations were underway. Women are told where to go but have to find their own way. They may be accompanied by a relative or friend but not by a member of staff. It is easy to get lost. The waiting room is normally busy and offers little privacy. If a woman is distressed attempts will be made to find a vacant curtained cubicle where she can compose herself but one is not always available. After the scan the women return to see the SHO in A&E for further discussion and arrangements for admission to hospital are made.

There are two experienced sonographers, one a superintendent, who undertake all the pregnancy scanning. They work under pressure. Ideally, ten minutes are allowed for a scan of this kind but often it is less than five. They describe themselves as a supportive team, confident in their skills and respected by their medical colleagues but feel isolated as practitioners, in their words 'in a world unto themselves'. They are concerned that they get no feedback on their work (did the woman understand the explanation that was given?) and lack knowledge about what happens to women before and after the scan. For example, the sonographers were unaware that it would be unusual for a woman diagnosed as miscarrying not to have an ERPC; they thought the purpose of the scan was to clarify whether one was necessary. They also incorrectly assumed that women routinely had the opportunity to talk about the miscarriage to other professionals.

The sonographers' task is to give a clear explanation of what the scan reveals in a language the woman can understand, questioning her to check her grasp of the information given. The sonographers routinely show women the screen and discuss the result with them. Partners are freely involved if they are present. They are concerned they may be patronising but are anxious to communicate well, as one of them describes:

> I know what it is like – if I go somewhere and I am not used to the surroundings or the terminology that people talking to me are using... then I don't take everything in... especially if you're full of emotions... which is why I do try and say 'Have you understood what I said? Do you want me to repeat it?'

The sonographers are aware that women often do not hear what is said to them but also that they remember in great detail how they are told and can be as upset by insensitivity as by the news itself. They try to pick up on the words a woman uses to talk about her pregnancy using the word 'baby' if she does.

Women's experiences

> They were very nice about the way they said it. Because they like speak in their sort of language if you know what I mean, like all these long words. And they said you know we'll write a letter and if you wait outside we'll send you back upstairs. Lots of tears.   Katy

> I could see the baby straight away. It was all curled up. It did look really nice... I wasn't really listening because I was looking at the baby... I was thinking... everything's fine. And then I can remember David [partner] was crying and I thought what has gone wrong and I started to listen. She was prodding to try and make the baby move and it wasn't moving. They told me that... due to how long my pregnancy was and how tall the fetus was they thought it had been dead for a while.   Carol

> I'm looking at the screen thinking well I can't see anything. I mean I don't know where I'm supposed to be looking but to me – when I first got in the picture of the woman before was still on the screen, she was

obviously quite far gone but you could see the baby and everything – and then there was me and I can't see anything, not a thing. And then she says I'm sorry to have to tell you this but I can't see anything, I think you have actually miscarried. Val

However much the women had been prepared for bad news by the GP or SHO, or because of the symptoms they experienced, it was at the scan when they fully realised that their pregnancy had failed (see Table 2.4). It was not always the words that conveyed the information. For Carol it was seeing the expression on her partner's face; for Pauline seeing the screen was important, as she describes:

It was just a natural explanation of what was going on. She wanted to show me... It helped me an awful lot seeing the empty sac... So it helped seeing something that wasn't dead, if you like. There was just nothing there.

All four women scanned at the hospital (one was not scanned and another was scanned elsewhere) described the scan as well handled. Despite the poor facilities and that Val saw the picture of the previous woman's well-formed baby on the screen when she went into the room, they valued highly the sensitivity and competence of the staff, the clear explanations they gave, the opportunity to see the screen and the involvement of their partners when present. The staff were described as 'really nice', approachable, understanding and sympathetic, and were remembered clearly by the women, who referred to them by their first name.

It is hard for staff working in these circumstances to do anything other than take what the women say at face value. For example, Pauline was on her own and devastated by the news, which she had not expected. She said it was the worst thing that had ever happened to her and the walk back to the A&E department from the scan the loneliest walk ever; she didn't know how she got there. However, she appeared calm, competent and in control. The sonographer was not concerned that she was alone and, even if she had been, would have been unable to do much about it.

The scan, when the miscarriage is confirmed, is a central part of the hospital experience and these sonographers underestimated the great personal significance they have to the women. Their importance to the women can perhaps be explained not only by the nature of the task and the personal qualities and skills of the sonographers but also by the brief nature of the contact women have with other staff when they miscarry. It is interesting to note that the sonographers as individuals and the scan as an event were of far more significance to the women who miscarried than to the women whose pregnancies were terminated at later gestations owing to an abnormality. In contrast, for these later women, the scan was the beginning of a lengthy episode of health care during which the women had the opportunity to develop a close relationship with nursing or midwifery staff. However, for the sonographers scanning women with suspected abnormalities was far more stressful and demanding than scanning women to confirm an early miscarriage.

❏ The SHO

Role of the SHO

Women will see the SHO on arrival in A&E, when they will be examined, a history taken and referral made to the ultrasound department. In theory women may have contact with the SHO on the emergency ward but, apart from Ann, who went straight to the ward, these women did not. The women took the high standard of medical care for granted and did not question in any way the medical competence of the staff who cared for them. The dimension in which the descriptions of their care differed was in the response to their emotional needs.

The SHOs are only too aware of the constraints under which they work – the lack of time, the pressure of numbers of people to be seen, the lack of privacy in A&E, the need to deal with the immediate crisis if the bleeding is heavy or the pain acute – but there is also some tension in their role. An experienced SHO recognised that a doctor's job was usually to make things better, to be a 'Mr Fix-it' but that you could not make it better for miscarriage patients although you could 'minimise the damage'. He identified two aspects to his role:

> I look at it two ways, it's the technical medicine bit where you make the diagnosis, you do the operation and you get them home... but then there's the emotional bit... Sure sometimes people don't want you to get involved but then that's their choice. At least they know that you are available if they want to talk.

In practice the SHOs differed in their views about how much their role extended beyond the medical examination and assessment and how far they should or could respond to the emotional aspects of miscarriage. An SHO who had only been in the job a few weeks describes his contact with Katy, who had a history of pregnancy loss. He clearly felt he ought to have offered more:

> I saw her very quickly in casualty because unfortunately there is great pressure over time when we see these ladies and it's far from ideal especially someone with her sort of background. She has obviously had a week at least to think about things and she was anxious and she wanted to talk... But it is always terribly busy and the pressure to see all these people in a short space of time, to get them in to have their scans which there is a deadline for. So we probably didn't talk very

much and you always feel you ought to be... doing a bit more counselling at that stage.

Katy felt that nobody talked to her or understood what it was like for her.

A more experienced SHO thought it appropriate to respond on an emotional level, to talk to women in some depth and had the confidence and skills to do so. He describes his approach:

I... just talked to her and asked her how she felt. I don't think I do ask that if I know that I haven't got time... Not everybody wants to talk but you are asking them to say how they are feeling. If you are just going to cut them off and just say well, 'I've got to go... I'm only giving you a minute', I think that's really unfair... If you know that you haven't got patients coming after this then you can and you can say something like 'How do you feel about this? What do you think has happened?' before you tell them what has happened. And usually that's when they probably start crying and that's when you can give them a hug then and spend time with them.

This contrasts with another SHO who cared for Laura. She was very focused in her task and thought the opportunity for discussion between doctor and patient in the A&E department limited and that the nurses on the ward were very good at talking to the women:

There just isn't the time... it's not the time and the place to go and sit and talk about it all. You're very much dealing with the acute situation of how we were going to stop the bleeding and stop the pain... the other things like loss tends to hit them a bit later.

Women may not want, or circumstances may prevent, discussion but clearly, as the above examples illustrate, the skill, experience, confidence and attitudes of the SHO will colour the service they as individuals offer women. The SHOs develop the skills of communicating with women about their miscarriage on the job. Several stressed the fact that, apart from a brief induction on the medical aspects of miscarriage, they had no training and acknowledged the lack of clarity over what they should say to women. As a new SHO summed up:

Nobody has ever taught me theoretically what I should say, or what ground we should cover with a lady that comes in with a known miscarriage. So I answer their questions as best as I can.

Explaining the miscarriage

A major part of the SHO's role is to explain the miscarriage as fully as possible although all the staff the women encounter contribute to their understanding of the miscarriage. One professional clearly builds on the work of another: the sonographer picking up on the seeds of doubt that they hope are sown by the GP and the SHO; the SHO confirming the scan result; GPs, anaesthetists, surgeons (registrars) and theatre and emergency nurses answering questions as they arise. However, the women in this study had more opportunity to discuss the miscarriage with the SHO than with any other health professional and clearly perceived this as part of the SHO's job.

All the women reported that they were given a clear explanation at the diagnosis of the miscarriage, were given information about procedures and were well prepared for what was going to happen to them, this being done sensitively. They described the SHOs as sympathetic, kind and caring. Pauline particularly valued the sensitivity of the SHO, who not only explained the miscarriage in ways she could understand but also acknowledged how she felt about it:

> He was very sympathetic really and very understanding which made me feel better. It made me feel all weepy when people are nice to you all the time... he explained it all medically as well. And he did it all just holding my hand all the time... I don't think I could have gone to anyone better than him really.

In contrast Val felt that although the SHO, who was new to the post, was caring in general terms he was unsympathetic about her pregnancy, which contributed to her sense of alienation and the feeling that nobody understood what she was going through:

> He was very nice but he knew... the pregnancy was wanted and he knew after we met that I had lost it and I just thought it would have been nice if he had said, 'I'm sorry to hear that you have lost it.' Instead of saying we'll have to send you up for a D&C... ignoring the fact that I had been pregnant in the first place... just being business-like about it.

Acknowledging the emotional reality of the pregnancy, that the reason women are seeking help is to do with a pregnancy and not some form of general illness, is particularly important for many women, who find miscarriage an intangible experience and afterwards begin to wonder whether they were ever pregnant. Some women may like to ignore the reality of the pregnancy, although none of the women in this study took that view, even though one had an appointment with her GP to request a termination of pregnancy and another had seriously considered it.

It is difficult for health professionals to know how women feel about it, and women may not know themselves, but it is generally accepted that it is usually most helpful to women to be honest and straightforward in the explanations given. An SHO acknowledged that 'when there isn't an awful lot to see' it is easy to forget that 'a lot of patients think "This is my baby."' A registrar describes how he explains a blighted ovum to women:

> I would tell her that there was no baby essentially... Something went very wrong early on in the pregnancy and, although the placenta was developed no baby, no fetus was actually beginning to develop and that perhaps was why the pregnancy wasn't continued on... So I would sort of play down, very much play down that it was a pregnancy and sort of swing her towards the idea that all she had... you know there had been a sort of a fertilisation of the egg but there wasn't anything there. I think, I don't know, I think sometimes it helps people accept things more, that there was something wrong.

Understanding that there is something wrong is important but emphasising the physical reality at the expense of the emotional reality is unlikely to be helpful and is likely to leave the woman confused.

There is a distinction between explanation and information about symptoms and procedures, and an explanation of the reasons for miscarriages. Two of the women clearly continued to be concerned about why miscarriages occur and why it had happened to them, as Laura describes:

> All they really gave me was this [booklet] which is... explaining not to worry about the miscarriage, I mean no-one really said why it happened, they just asked me 'was it planned?' – the pregnancy – and sorry to hear about it really. You know everyone was very apologetic. I mean no-one actually sat down and said why.

Once out of hospital it may be difficult for women to get this information.

❏ **Communication about the remains of the pregnancy**

Information about the remains of the pregnancy: women's views

> A lot of women just don't ask. They don't want to know or they're too frightened. They don't know how to ask. The doctors don't allow open questions.   GP

Perhaps the dilemmas the SHO faces in communicating with women are best illustrated in talking about the physical nature of the loss. Communication about the remains of the pregnancy, whether it be products of conception or complete embryo, was universally difficult for women and staff.

Although the women varied in their knowledge of the physical development of their pregnancy they were aware of the changes taking place in their body, aware of the developing pregnancy and thought of their pregnancy, to a greater or lesser extent, in terms of a baby (see Table 2.3). Consequently, when they miscarried they expected there to be a physical loss and were concerned about its nature.

Only Pauline, who was described by the sonographer as having a 'textbook blighted ovum' and who interpreted this as 'there was nothing there and nothing to worry about', was unconcerned about this aspect of her care. The remaining five women were left with unanswered questions ranging from concern that large clots they had lost were in fact the baby, to ignorance, because no-one had seen fit to tell them about what was removed at the ERPC and there was no opportunity to ask. None of these women were concerned at seeing the loss, including the woman who had seen a complete fetus on the screen at her scan and who said she wished to keep that as her memory, but all wanted to know about it. None of the women reported asking questions at the time, either because they did not feel able to or it did not occur to them. These are questions to which it is very hard to get answers after the event.

Laura's experience

Laura's experience illustrates the complexity of this issue. She was bleeding heavily and was attended by an SHO in A&E. She was concerned about the remains of the pregnancy:

> The only thing I did see which she put into this pot were two great big clots about the size of ping pong balls and she put them over on the side with some things and she saw me looking at them. She said, 'They're clots that I have taken away to send to analyse', but she didn't actually show them to me and say, 'Look this is what has come out of you'. I mean I was actually looking at them... It was quite a shock... She did say, 'Are there any questions you want to ask?' but at that time I didn't. But in a way it was the way she... put it over... And she only explained because she saw me looking at them... I think all the time I was bleeding I was waiting for something to come out. Almost like going through pregnancy I suppose... She just said at the end, 'Yes, you've had a miscarriage and you will be going for your D&C where you have to be cleaned out... The clots, they're being sent off.' At the time... I just thought well where do they go? What will the results be and how will I know? Because to me as far as I'm concerned I've had my D&C, they've taken the clots and I'm no longer anybody. That's how I feel... You know when things are taken from you, you do want to know but she didn't say, 'Well you can contact your GP to find out the results or if you want to come back here'... None of that was explained.

The SHO had in fact removed the sac with a complete embryo but referred to it as a clot and put it in a jar on the side 'to save the woman's feelings'. Based on her previous experience she thought it would be insensitive to explain what it was and feared Laura's reaction if she did as she described:

> The women I've had who... have passed a sac on their own or passed clots have been really upset and absolutely freaked out that they've seen it and I've had to say I'm not sure. I think sometimes it is enough to say that the pregnancy is over rather than say this is it I'm going to pop it in a pot now. I'm not sure that there is necessarily a lot to be gained by seeing it... I'm not sure it particularly helped them.

Laura had a clear image in her mind of what had been removed and wondered if 'the clots were her baby'. She was still wondering when interviewed and will probably never find out.

Professional responsibility

For relatively inexperienced SHOs this is a difficult issue to deal with. Not only may they lack the confidence in what to say and how to handle the situation sensitively but women vary in what they want to know as well as in their ability to ask. In Laura's case she was given the opportunity to ask questions but at the time 'didn't get it together' to do so. It is clear from the SHO's account that Laura would have needed to be direct and unemotional in her questions to get an accurate answer. It seems unrealistic to place the responsibility on women to take the initiative in this way.

An experienced GP, who had herself miscarried as well as cared for a lot of patients post-miscarriage, argued that health professionals must be proactive. She thought it a professional responsibility, specifically the SHO's, to create the opportunity for women to ask questions and to provide information about the remains of the pregnancy:

> You're vulnerable, you're emotional. You can't ask anything; you don't think to ask anything. You just think 'I must be a good patient. I'll lie here and not say anything.' And you [the doctor] need to be aware of those issues to bring them up to deal with them. You can't leave it for the patient to bring up those issues, because they won't. Particularly the inarticulate patients. You [the interviewer] might, I might, probably I wouldn't even... Not when you're vulnerable without your knickers and stuck on a trolley somewhere.

She went on to describe how she thought this should be done, stressing that it was not up to the staff to decide on a woman's behalf what was acceptable or not and that women would differ in their views:

If you're removing a clot from someone you need to say, 'This is just a clot of blood. There isn't any baby here to see.' Or if there is... you need to say, 'the baby is here, would you like to see the baby?' And sometimes that's important... If it was me I would like to see it. Now some would say, 'Oh no no no take it away.'

It is only recently that this would have been considered acceptable practice and not all health professionals will share her views. Some may have strong personal reactions and find the products of conception, embryo or fetus repulsive in some way, so be unable to handle the matter in the straightforward manner proposed by the GP quoted above. An SHO had assisted in theatre during an operation to remove an ectopic pregnancy when a complete embryo was removed. He describes the differing reactions of staff and patient:

It was eight weeks and it had little fingers, little legs... he [registrar] put it in a pot, separated it away from the blood. We kept that to show, if the woman wanted to see it. And apparently last night, her husband did see it and he took some pictures of it... She wasn't awake apparently... but she had photos. So it was important for him as well. I thought that was a brilliant idea... We were all amazed... It looked so lovely because it was in its whole sac as well and there was fluid in the sac... But when the sister put it in the pot – somebody who was helping label it was saying, 'That's really gross. That's really disgusting. Why do you want to show her that? I wouldn't want to see it.' I was thinking well in some ways some people might think it's horrible but if you've got it there in a nice clean pot and it's clear and at least you can say do you want to or not.

❏ **Disposal**

Women's views

Disposal was not an issue for the women in this study. They wondered what had been removed during the ERPC or about the nature of the physical loss (clots, tissue etc.) but were unconcerned about what happened to it.

Hospital policy

It is the policy of the hospital in this study to package the products of each conception individually. The remains are checked in the pathology department for confirmation of pregnancy, infection and evidence of a molar pregnancy. They are stored and on a weekly basis incinerated separately from other hospital waste at another hospital some distance away. Following the suction termination of pregnancy the products are not packaged separately but strained and collected together in a Sharps' box.

Health professionals' views

Apart from the consultant obstetricians most of the junior doctors (registrars and SHOs) had inadequate knowledge and understanding about the handling and disposal of the remains of the pregnancy following early miscarriage. Except for those who had personal experience of miscarriage the GPs were similarly ill informed. Ignorance about common practice meant they would have been unable to answer questions accurately if asked. Many said they had not thought about it much before being interviewed for this research. Like this experienced SHO they were unable to answer the questions we asked:

> Well as far as I know they just get sent to the lab and then they are
> put in formalin. Basically they just make sure... I don't know actually.
> After the lab's finished with them I have no idea.

It was the general view that women did not ask questions about the disposal of products of conception. Few said they had any experience of being asked although one of the consultants commented that he thought more women who miscarried were asking now because it was acceptable to do so and that questions in this area would increase. It was generally thought that women were not concerned about disposal and that information would cause additional distress. The possible emotional importance for women was not acknowledged. Several of the hospital doctors who were aware of changing attitudes expressed strong views about the inappropriateness of complicated disposal arrangements following a miscarriage, questioning whose benefit it was for, that 'burial or cremation for first trimester loss was over the top'. The GPs with personal experience of miscarriage thought this was perfectly acceptable if that was what women wanted but that not many would.

Concern about the acceptability of the procedures, and in consequence fear of women's reactions if they knew, was common. One registrar commented that he was very glad women did not ask about this as it would be very awkward. Another who had experience of patients asking about what happens to the early remains said he tells them as delicately as he can but is aware he fudges it. He made the comparison with the inaccurate information doctors give about post mortems and explained this in terms of a lack of knowledge on the doctor's part about what is involved and a lack of understanding about why women might be asking. One GP said he would lie if a woman asked about what happened to her fetus from an early miscarriage. Ignorance about the system and concern about the acceptability of procedures he thought to be in operation combined to make it difficult for this SHO to communicate honestly with his patient:

It's very difficult to reassure people that what has been taken away which they may or may not think of as their baby depending on their views of when life begins... the tissue is... treated with the respect that you would offer to a stillborn baby for instance... I suspect that it is just treated as clinical waste like... something that has been removed during an operation... I'm not sure I wouldn't be tempted to lie actually to make a... I mean I would think of it as a white lie...

The nurses on the emergency ward also lacked accurate knowledge. They knew that 'it goes to the lab' but not much beyond that. Even though they did not know what they were, there was a general feeling that hospital procedures 'were good enough'. Most of the nurses stressed that they were never asked, the implication being that it was only a problem if women themselves were concerned. One suggested that it was easier for women the less they knew. Several nurses linked women's need to know about disposal with the gestation of the pregnancy. One said she only thought it was a problem after about 16 weeks of pregnancy when there was a recognisable fetus and another that when women miscarried early in pregnancy they did not see it as a baby so it was not a problem.

Discussion about disposal after an early miscarriage is clearly an issue that few if any of the staff these women encountered could have handled competently and honestly owing to a lack of basic information about procedures, a lack of understanding of the potential importance for women and the emotional process the women might be going through, personal distaste at the procedures and concern about their acceptability to women, or fear of women's reactions if they knew. Ignorance about the system may protect staff from having to answer questions about something they find disturbing or distasteful. Women may not ask questions because in subtle ways staff communicate that it is not to be talked about.

❏ Inpatient care

Emergency ward

In this hospital women requiring an ERPC are admitted to the emergency ward. It is a 32-bedded unit with a high turnover of patients. Up to 16 admissions per day is not unusual. It is estimated that at any one time there are usually four patients on the ward who have miscarried or have an ectopic pregnancy. The ward consists of some side rooms and a series of six- to eight-bedded units. Attempts are always made to put the women who have miscarried or who have ectopic pregnancies together. The only privacy that is available is that afforded by pulling the curtains around the bed. Some women who miscarry later in pregnancy or who have a termination for abnormality are occasionally cared for in the side rooms of this ward.

The emergency ward forms part of the chain of care for women who miscarry. Women will come to the ward from the A&E department, go down to theatre and return to the ward before discharge home. Tension between the emergency ward and the A&E department was acknowledged by some of the nurses particularly concerning nursing care and pain relief, which they considered were inadequately provided. In contrast the maternity unit was held in high regard and perceived as available to give advice when needed.

The ward is busy; many different consultants will have patients there. By definition the majority of patients require emergency treatment. Some patients are extremely ill, some die and it is common to have distressed relatives on the ward. In contrast to these patients, women who miscarry are not ill, are not generally considered to be an emergency and, as a consequence, come bottom of the priority list. It is generally recognised by the gynaecologists that this ward is not a good location for the care of miscarriage patients. It is too busy and the contrast with the other patients too marked.

The nursing staff say they enjoy caring for the miscarriage patients and would miss them if they were cared for elsewhere. However, several of the nurses recognised the difficulties of caring for women following an ERPC in an acute setting. The nurses feel very pressured, often unable to give women the time they feel they need. The nurses have limited knowledge of protocols and guidelines concerning the care of miscarriage patients and information is handed on from one nurse to another.

The ward is a demanding and stressful place to work but the nursing staff describe themselves as members of a stable and supportive, ward-based team; they feel they can turn to each other for help when they need it. There is a great deal of respect for the leadership and guidance offered by the sister in charge. The nurses who cared for the women in this study were all quite young, two being student nurses.

Women who felt well cared for

Pauline, Laura and Carol felt well cared for on the emergency ward and appreciated the high standard of nursing care. The ward was relatively quiet during their hospital admission. They all described the nurses as friendly and helpful, and gave detailed examples of incidents when they felt particularly well cared for. In their relatively short time on the ward they clearly felt that a nurse or nurses engaged with them. For example, Carol, who bled very heavily after the ERPC and 'was really worried about dirtying everything up', was very grateful for the way the nurse cleaned her up and helped her get back to bed.

Laura, who arrived on the ward in the middle of the night bleeding heavily and in pain, appreciated the sensitivity and acceptance of the nursing staff:

She went and organised that [painkiller] very quickly and then she explained that I had another one [injection] to stop me being sick. That was it really but she was just so pleasant. She just made me feel I was OK. She just made me feel quite comfortable… She said I would be going up to have my D&C the next day and just made sure I was warm enough and if I needed anything.

The nurse caring for her was clear that Laura was upset and just wanted to get the pain settled and go to sleep. When she returned to the ward after the ERPC she valued the lack of questioning of the day staff and their friendly and helpful attitude:

Nothing was too much trouble. She was in and out every five minutes just checking you know. 'Would you like some food?' 'Are you in pain?' And she said about me going home and I said, 'I haven't got any money, I can't phone my boyfriend' and she said, 'Well would you like me to?'… It was almost as if she'd known us ages… She was there all the time and very light, 'Hi, you OK?' That sort of attitude.

These women did not want to talk at length about their situation but said there was sufficient opportunity to talk to the nurses. They valued the explanations they were given of different procedures and their questions were answered although, at the time, they did not have many. They did not want the nurses to probe and wanted to keep communication on a fairly superficial level; as Pauline said, 'The nurses were nice and chatty and kept my mind off it'.

Women who described the care as poor

Similarly, Katy, Val and Ann, who were critical of their care, reported that the nurses were friendly and kind but also that they were unable to give them the attention they needed. They said no-one really talked to them and their feelings were not acknowledged. They described the nurses as 'nice but they had no time', and the ward as 'very busy' and the nurses as 'rushed off their feet'. The nurses agreed. But the women also described situations in which they clearly felt let down, of not getting things they had been promised: a member of staff who they had been told would come and talk to them, the telephone, food and their buzzer left unanswered. In addition they all reported muddles about their blood (blood sample lost, confusion about their blood group or persistent and repetitive questions about it) which served to undermine their confidence in their medical care. They all thought other patients were more important because they were seriously ill and 'you're not that ill with a miscarriage'. In short they felt neglected.

Katy and Ann, who had a history of pregnancy loss, described the staff as 'not understanding', 'they haven't been through it', and 'keeping their distance'. The nurses thought these women 'didn't need much because they'd been through it all before' and 'they knew the ropes'. Katy said she did not have much to do with the nurses 'not to have a conversation, they're too busy'. She thought the nurse was more interested in her young daughter, who was visiting, than in her. She described the nurses as 'useless at answering questions because they didn't know anything' and was resentful that when the nurses did talk to her it was only to ask her questions she thought they should know the answers to:

> The thing that annoys me is – well they didn't know what blood group I was. I mean they only have to look at your notes and they know... And they should know what happened last time. They shouldn't have to come and ask me again. Like she said, 'How far gone was you last time when you lost it?' And I thought, 'Oh no.' And it should be on my notes. I mean they only have to look at the notes and they know... They didn't even know that I was supposed to have a stitch or I've got a weak cervix.

Val only spent three hours on the emergency ward after the ERPC and was disenchanted with her care before she got there. There was a delay of more than two hours in transferring her from the recovery room to the ward. She describes her experience of waking up in the recovery room aware that other people were seriously ill:

> I woke up and I started to cry... It seemed more final then, somehow, when I'd had this D&C. And they just kept walking past me all the time sort of looking at me. One woman came over and said, 'Are you OK?' and I said 'Yeah' and off they went again, doing other things. And a couple were chatting over here and I'm just laying there crying. I just wanted to... I didn't really want to be there. I'd rather be on the ward than be in there... I felt the whole time that everything was more important than me and so I shouldn't make a fuss.

Sadly, the nurse caring for her in recovery was sympathetic and aware of her plight but did not talk to her, assuming that the nurse on the emergency ward would do so. On the emergency ward the nurse only came to talk to her when her mother requested help because she thought her daughter needed counselling before she went home. Val compared her care unfavourably with her care when she had an abortion at a private abortion clinic:

> They weren't unfriendly. They were nice but I just got fed up with hearing that same line [miscarriage is very common]. And just one person to say, 'Are you all right? Sorry to hear the bad news.' Just somebody to hold your hand. There was nothing like that. I mean... when I had an abortion... when I came to I had someone with me

giving me a lot more sympathy... and I didn't even want that. But when I actually wanted one I didn't get anything.

Nurses' views

Nurses on the emergency ward are responsible for admitting women to the ward, preparing them for the ERPC and caring for them postoperatively. The nurses described the different aspects of their task in admitting women who miscarry to the ward: take their history, check their physical health, explain the procedures and prepare them for the ERPC. In addition they considered it important to listen to the women, to give them information, to enable them to ask questions and to show they cared.

Caring for women prior to the ERPC, particularly if they are bleeding heavily, can be distressing especially, as one nurse said, if 'there is little you can do except give them pads'. A nurse describes her role in caring for Laura prior to the ERPC. She thought her role more limited owing to the constraints of night duty:

I just try and be there really. So the next thing you see of them apart from checking during the night that they're asleep, they're OK, is the next morning when you do the temperature and antibiotics if they need any and just say, 'Are you all right? Do you need anything?'

A day nurse describes her role in caring for Pauline after she returned from theatre:

to make sure that she wasn't in pain, make sure she wasn't bleeding a lot after the operation, make sure that there weren't any complications there, make sure she herself was all right. If she wanted to know whether she could eat or drink. Inform her of what the procedure was postop so that she could go home as soon as possible... Making sure she understands what went on down there, what she can expect when she goes home.

The time most women spend on the ward is short and characterised by anxiety about the operation or drowsiness afterwards. All the nurses stressed how busy the ward gets at times and how impossible it can be to spend a lot of time with the miscarriage patients as one nurse described:

It's so difficult in such a short space of time because they're literally here only for a few hours. You have to get them ready and organised quickly as well and they are probably here on the ward for an hour and a half and then they're downstairs... They come back and they're here for a couple of hours, sleeping, and then they go home... We can only devote so much time because you've got to prioritise all the other things you've got to do as well which I think on the whole the women understand.

The nurses clearly rely on the women to ask questions or to indicate that they want to talk or need more than basic help. One nurse described how she handled it:

Usually I say, 'How do you feel about things?' and quite often they say, 'I'm all right.' And then it's hard... you can't really probe any more than that... I usually say, 'Well if you want to talk or anything, you do know I'm here all afternoon', so they can always come back to me later on... I feel you can't probe too much because it's a very personal thing... I think they would have asked if they wanted to, if they had a problem. Also I don't think someone has time to adjust... in hospital... I don't think they have time to absorb it all.

The nurses were concerned about what to say to women, stressing the importance of 'choosing questions carefully so that women don't feel you're prying into their life' and how much to probe. They expressed reservations about the appropriateness of talking to women when they are in hospital, in crisis and physically unwell, the unsuitability of the emergency ward, too busy and lacking in privacy, and the lack of time. Interestingly, it is often the student nurses who are allocated to women who miscarry because they have more time. Yet they are less skilled in talking with women about their feelings, have less knowledge about the system of care and a less developed understanding of miscarriage, perhaps resorting more easily to factual questions about the woman's history or everyday chat.

Discomfort in handling women's distress was a common theme in nurses' accounts of their care of miscarriage patients. One described how difficult she found women who were overtly upset:

It just very much depends on their attitude. I don't think I'm very good with weeping and wailing women. But I think ones that are a bit more practical and realistic... I find easier to relate to... I mean I don't think I'm any less sympathetic but it's very hard to find the right words to comfort somebody if I've never experienced that sort of problem.

Clearly, the service that it is possible to offer within the constraints of the emergency ward suits women such as Pauline, Laura and Carol but not those like Katy, Val or Ann. They needed time and staff who could reach out to them and who were comfortable with handling the complexity of their reactions whether fuelled by ignorance, confusion and shock as in Val's case or by the deeper despair of infertility as in Ann's.

It is assumed by the sonographers and some of the junior doctors that the emergency ward is where women have the opportunity 'to talk if they want to' and where 'the nursing staff are very good' but from the experience of women in this study it is clear that it does not happen. Women can pass through the hospital system of care having had very little personal contact with any member of staff even though they wanted it. They feel no-one has connected with them or understood their situation and they have unanswered questions. The staff of the emergency ward find comfort in the fact that women are told to go to their GP, the health visitor is always informed and women are given information about the self-help groups, thus having ample opportunities to get further help should they need it.

Discharge from hospital

> The only thing they did explain was that I would probably still bleed for ten days and if after that there was any problems I was supposed to go and see my GP. But that is all I remember them telling me. But the rest of the information I got from that booklet... They just let me go from the hospital and that was it really. I suppose they feel I'm old enough and big enough to do whatever. Laura

On discharge women should be given a booklet which includes information about the causes of miscarriage, likely physical and emotional reactions and sources of further help. They are also advised to make an appointment with their GP in a couple of weeks time but to seek more immediate help from their GP or from A&E should the bleeding increase. The GP and health visitor should be informed of the miscarriage and antenatal appointments cancelled.

All the women described their discharge from the emergency ward in negative terms:

> It was a long wait to see a different doctor who then didn't do anything and didn't even introduce himself.

> I was given no information.

> There was no discussion with a doctor.

> The nurses were too busy to talk.

> I had to ask if I could go.

The discharge procedure was clearly contrary to women's expectations that something significant would happen to release them from the hospital. They described it as an 'anticlimax', 'a non-event' and 'abrupt'. There was little discussion about going home and how they might feel in the next few days and, if they were given the opportunity to ask questions, they clearly didn't feel able to. Only three of the women were given the leaflet, which all said they found useful in the absence of anything else.

■ After discharge from hospital

❑ GP care

GP's role

A duty to support and assist in any way I can.   GP

Providing follow-up care after a miscarriage was viewed by these GPs as an important but not particularly demanding part of their work. The GPs included in their tasks dealing with any physical problems, providing information and explanation as well as 'being available' to offer support to women and their partners when they needed it, which may not be until some time later. The more experienced GPs stressed the importance of 'keeping an open door', of enabling women to come back at any time, aware that many women did not want 'to be pestered early on'.

All the GPs interviewed were critical of the service the hospital provided in terms of meeting women's needs whilst realistic in their expectations of what could be offered, understanding the constraints under which the hospital operated. They were therefore aware of the potential importance of their role. One GP described it as 'picking up the pieces afterwards', answering the questions that had arisen, explaining aspects of hospital care that remained puzzling and talking about the future if that was appropriate. Laura's GP describes how she approaches follow-up care:

> I just chat through their feelings really in the follow-up appointment. And they often have lots of questions, they don't understand why the baby died, they want to know if I know why the baby died, if they did anything wrong, was it something they had done, what were their chances of it happening again? That sort of thing, the sort of medical questions they ask. And then also I try and also explore with them their feelings about it and their tearfulness and their great sort of grief that they feel no-one really acknowledges around them and I actually try and verbalise it's OK to feel really down about it... It's normal and... they've lost a baby and it wasn't just a little blob that people have thought 'Oh well, it's just a miscarriage.' And I think verbalising helps them, just to say it's OK to grieve and that people understand and you're not alone in your feelings... Also to just talk through, often their partner's feelings, often the partner might not appreciate how down they are feeling and to talk about how long they might feel really very down for. And they often want to talk about when it is OK to try again and... well I would say they can start as soon as they want because there are a lot of myths around that you mustn't try for three months. There is no medical reason for that... I say when it is right for you, you go for it... And it's really just generally empathising with them and saying that you can come back, it's OK and you're not abnormal in the way you feel.

Laura's GP was confident and comfortable in approaching the emotional aspects of miscarriage. A trainee GP was more cautious, fearing she would intrude on a woman's personal privacy, as she describes:

> I'm not even sure it's our role to get deep into all this because some people will like to be supported by their family and their friends and they've got other support mechanisms and I think it's maybe almost encroaching into their personal space and what they want.

The more experienced GPs acknowledged the difficulty of identifying those women who are strongly affected by the miscarriage and were more confident about initiating contact with women and broaching what might be considered sensitive subjects.

Women's views

The women's health care needs following their discharge from hospital differed. Table 2.7 summarises the nature of the contact the women had with their GP and the women's and GPs' views about it. The women who had a GP they identified as their doctor and who did not have to initiate the contact with the GP after the miscarriage when they felt vulnerable were more positive about their care.

Pauline, Laura, Katy and Carol, all of whom had a GP they called 'their own', already had an appointment or their GP had suggested they make one after the miscarriage. Their GPs were involved with their care and concerned about their well-being, communicating this to the women. The contact women had with their GP varied. For Pauline a telephone call was sufficient. Laura did not keep the appointment that had been made. Carol was critical of her GP's emphasis on the physical as opposed to the psychological despite the GP describing her role as 'someone to cry to'. Nevertheless the woman did not have to initiate the contact.

Despite the objectively good-quality follow-up care offered to Katy, whose GP gave her a lot of time, took the trouble to contact her and made sure she had full information and opportunities to discuss the miscarriage, she eventually appeared to reject his help. Her reasons for doing this appear to be due to criticisms of his off-hand manner and a feeling that 'he was no longer on her side'. Following what was her second miscarriage she was very sensitive and vulnerable. She changed to a different GP at the practice: 'a woman who would understand'.

Val and Ann, neither of whom had a GP they identified as 'their doctor', were critical of their care. Both had anxieties about their physical health after the miscarriage. Ann had an adverse reaction to the anaesthetic, which frightened her and necessitated a home visit by the GP. Over the next few months she had several visits to the GP surgery for treatment for a recurrent vaginal infection. Her infertility and miscarriage were not discussed. Val

Table 2.7 Early miscarriage: health care after discharge from hospital

	GP care	Women's views	GPs' views	Other professional help
Pauline*	telephone call from GP shortly after her return home	telephone call appreciated and sufficient	a capable woman who was distressed by the miscarriage; will offer support in next pregnancy	–
Laura*	follow-up appointment with GP made but not kept	–	will wait for Laura to contact her	–
Katy	telephone call from GP and several appointments to check her well-being, both physical and psychological, and to discuss future pregnancy	critical of GPs' informal manner; changed GP to a 'woman who would understand'	gave a lot of time and support; did best in the circumstances	–
Carol	several appointments with the GP for contraception and smear; GP referred to practice counsellor	GP concentrated on physical well-being and medical care, not psychological which she considered the purpose of appointment	thought it important that GP is 'available to cry to' after the miscarriage	GP referred to practice counsellor; unsatisfactory so private counselling help sought
Val	appointment with GP due to concern with post-miscarriage bleeding	unsatisfactory; symptoms not taken seriously; changed GP	not interviewed	in desperation attended Well Woman clinic at the surgery where the practice nurse was very helpful in sharing her own experience of miscarriage
Ann	home visit and two appointments due to problems post-miscarriage following anaesthetic and then recurring vaginal infection	each time saw a different GP, all unsympathetic, 'don't understand infertility'; changed GP	not interviewed	telephone call from nurse at hospital where treated for infertility, helpful; telephone call to practice nurse at GP surgery with whom had contact during pregnancy

* No second interview with woman so information limited.

was concerned about the extent of bleeding and needed medical reassurance as well as the opportunity to talk about the miscarriage, which she felt she did not get:

> I waited and waited in the waiting room and when I got through it was a woman doctor who obviously didn't know anything that had gone on so I had to explain everything again... I had started bleeding... which I didn't think I was supposed to do after they'd done a D&C. So she just said, 'Is it heavy?' And I said, 'Well it's not heavy'. 'So it's mild then?' 'No it's not mild then either it's just in between.' She said, 'Well if it continues you'll have to come back and we'll put you on a course of antibiotics.'

The lack of effective involvement and support from their GPs echoed the disjointed and personally disconnected care both these women had experienced in hospital. They complained of the unsympathetic treatment by the GP; they saw a different doctor at each consultation; their symptoms were trivialised; the loss of miscarriage and infertility was misunderstood. In desperation Val attended the Well Woman clinic because she wanted 'to check that everything was all right' and found the practice nurse, whom she discovered had experienced miscarriage herself, extremely helpful to talk to. Both women changed to a different GP for their future health care.

❑ Further support

These women felt well supported by their partner, family (particularly mother and sisters) or a friend. They had people to talk to about the miscarriage and none of the women contacted the voluntary self-help group (the Miscarriage Association). They said they did not need this sort of help, they did not like groups and it was not for them. They may have felt that some of the professionals or some of their friends or family lacked understanding but they did not feel alone and unable to share the experience with anyone. For them the miscarriage was not the hidden experience that many women have described in the past.

Women clearly differ in the extent of their own personal support networks and their need for and the use they would make of counselling help or support from a professional. Some of the GPs considered there were other people to take on this role if necessary: a health visitor or practice counsellor. None of these women was contacted by a health visitor although it is the local system that the health visitor should be informed. Only Katy, who already had a child, knew of her health visitor. Carol, who was clearly in crisis a few months after the miscarriage, was referred by her GP to the practice counsellor. She eventually sought counselling help privately as she was dissatisfied with the practice counsellor. She reported that appointments were infrequent and often cancelled.

Counselling help or further support from a professional was not routinely offered or widely available. Several of the women said they would have welcomed help had they been unable to get pregnant again and one woman was particularly concerned about her husband's reaction to her miscarriage and infertility. These women would have found it difficult to ask for further help if they needed it and would not have known where to get it.

❑ Women's reactions in the six months after discharge

Table 2.8 summarises the women's reactions over the six-month period of the project. Apart from Laura, who dropped out after the first interview, and Pauline, who maintained written and telephone contact for five months, the women remained with the project and completed the second interview. When considering the women's reactions over the six-month period it is helpful to distinguish between the women's reactions at the time of the miscarriage and their longer-term reactions over the following months. The time of the miscarriage was clearly a crisis for all the women regardless of their feelings about the pregnancy. Their reactions in subsequent months were, predictably, more varied. Feeling able to try again (for those who wished to be pregnant) was a turning point in the intervening months and getting pregnant another. Focus on a future pregnancy appeared to help the women and support them in their recovery.

Pauline, Katy and Val, once over the initial distress of the miscarriage, described themselves as 'getting on with it'. They made minor changes to their lives: Pauline changed to a less stressful job, Katy and Val improved their diet. They all described times when they got upset, often triggered by a specific event like a friend's pregnancy or a television programme, and how these lessened over time. Katy and Val became pregnant again quite quickly and Pauline was, at the last contact, hoping to be.

Two of the women appeared to be more seriously affected by the miscarriage. Ann was clearly very distressed after the miscarriage and, with her history of infertility, hopeless about ever having a child. She described herself as depressed and unwell for some time, rarely went out and was pessimistic about her future. Four months after the miscarriage she began to feel more positive and able to try again, her second chance at IVF. By the time of the second interview she was eight weeks pregnant, resting, hoping and trying not to get too excited.

At the time Carol described herself as 'putting a brave face on it' but her distress and turmoil came to a head about three months after the miscarriage when she described herself as unable to stop crying, unable to go out of the house and having recurring nightmares about pregnancy and fertility. Three months after this she was more philosophical, had sought counselling help and, although sad about the miscarriage, was relieved the pregnancy had not continued. For Carol the miscarriage represented a turning point in

Table 2.8 Early miscarriage: women's reactions in the six months after discharge

	Reactions at the time	In the intervening months	Six months after the miscarriage
Pauline*	had a 'weepy weekend' then back to normal	got on with life, 'just one of those things, happens to lot of people'; changed job and lifestyle	optimistic and trying again (diary sheet – five months after miscarriage)
Laura**	distress at trauma and pain; relief no longer pregnant	–	–
Katy	distress, reliving earlier miscarriages	dismissed the impact of this miscarriage as trivial compared with earlier experience; one month after miscarriage started trying again	miscarriage behind her; 20 weeks pregnant; feels well and optimistic
Carol	angry and distressed	'put a brave face on it', then crisis three months after miscarriage: crying, nightmares, felt she was 'going mad'	sad about the miscarriage but also relieved; continues to be distressed but, with counselling help, is sorting out personal issues to do with pregnancy, relationships and the direction of her life
Val	cried a lot in hospital	'felt sad but basically I got on with it'; occasional upset triggered by specific event, e.g. friend's pregnancy	ten weeks pregnant; feels well and optimistic
Ann	acutely distressed; felt ill	distressed and hopeless, crying, unable to do anything, physically unwell; began to get better four months after miscarriage and felt able to try again	eight weeks pregnant; 'in neutral', resting, hoping and trying not to get excited

* No second interview. Written contact for five months post-miscarriage.

** No contact after first interview.

her life when she was faced with, in her view, the irresponsible way she had been living her life and felt she had to grow up.

It was these two women who, in different ways, appeared to focus most on the miscarriage as the loss of a baby. Ann talked about this miscarriage and her previous two ectopic pregnancies: 'I know they weren't real babies but they were to me. I will always remember them, never forget.' She discussed doing something to remember the babies, possibly going to church to light a candle and to thank God for her present pregnancy, although she described herself as 'not a religious person'. Carol, who in her early pregnancy prior to the miscarriage had focused intensely on the baby, also thought it important to mark her baby's short life:

> I wrote him a letter. We both wrote a letter. We put them in a box and tied it up with ribbon. I suppose... I was more like angry than anything else. I was more shocked. But no I didn't keep anything else.

■ Conclusion

The ethos of care for the women who miscarry is that of a minor medical emergency at the bottom of the medical priority list to be promptly and efficiently dealt with. The hospital system determines that a miscarriage is considered a one-off event with no history and in no context. Care is compartmentalised, fragmented and often impersonal, and the stay in hospital short with little opportunity to talk about the emotional aspects of the miscarriage. Women are expected to take responsibility for themselves and take the initiative in asking for help or in making their needs known. Whilst this may suit some women it has grave limitations for women who do not view their miscarriage in this way, who have wider psychological needs or who are more passive and undemanding.

Women clearly vary in their experience and interpretation of their miscarriage and, in consequence, in the subtleties of the health care that is appropriate for them. Health professionals concerned with offering a high standard of care are then faced with the difficulties of understanding individual need, of making a rigid system of care more suitable for a variety of individuals and of the stresses and strains of working within a system which offers them little flexibility in doing so.

■ Issues in good practice arising from the research

❏ Staffing and training

These considerations are appropriate for all staff involved in the care of women who miscarry, particularly SHOs and nursing staff, but also GPs and sonographers.

The diversity of experience

The physical experience of the miscarriage and the women's reactions at the time and later varied from an event that was physically inconsequential, emotionally insignificant and could be viewed as a short-term crisis to an event that was medically significant and perceived as a major loss. The emotional reality of the miscarriage does not necessarily match the physical reality and is not neatly linked to gestation. The way a women felt about her miscarriage was affected by her personal history and characteristics as well as by her expectations and present circumstances. A set formula of care is therefore likely to fail many women. In order to offer effective care health professionals:

- need awareness of the diversity of experience
- should not make assumptions about the meaning or significance of the miscarriage or take a woman's reactions at face value
- should check out with a woman how she is feeling, what she wants to happen and what she wants to know.

Professional responsibility

The nurse, sonographer, gynaecologist and GP all play an important part in providing good care. A miscarriage is generally a crisis, distasteful and unexpected, for which women are unprepared, whilst health care is fragmented and contact with health professionals brief. Women are vulnerable and will not know what options they have. Professionals must therefore take responsibility for maximising a woman's opportunity for good care. In order to do this professionals must be proactive and take responsibility for:

- creating the opportunity for questions to be asked
- asking and anticipating questions
- raising difficult issues
- giving choice where this is possible
- having accurate knowledge, beyond the scope of their own input, of the strengths and limitations of the health care system for women who miscarry.

Handling the emotional aspects of miscarriage

The emotional aspects of miscarriage are often avoided by health professionals. The emotional significance of a miscarriage is not acknowledged and opportunities to talk about how a women feels are either not created or not taken. Staff often do not know what to say or fear intruding on a woman's privacy. It is frequently assumed that it is another professional's responsibility to talk about feelings. Ignoring the emotional aspects of miscarriage is generally unhelpful to women. Staff need to be able to acknowledge how a woman may be feeling and talk to her about it. This means good communication not lengthy counselling. Staff may be helped to do this through:

- knowledge of how women are likely to react
- understanding their own reactions
- developing skills and building confidence in talking with women.

Communication about the remains of the pregnancy

It is generally inaccurately assumed by health professionals that women are unconcerned about the nature of the remains of the pregnancy and, as it is distasteful and potentially upsetting, the subject is avoided. It should be assumed that women want to know unless they make it clear to the contrary. Many health professionals are ill informed about local policy and practice.

In order to provide women with the information they may want staff need:

- to develop the communication skills outlined above
- accurate information about the remains of a pregnancy and about the hospital's policy on disposal.

Feedback

Many health professionals complained that they never got any feedback on the way they approached a patient so worked in a vacuum. It was common for staff to underestimate their significance for women and the power inherent in their role as a professional. Many also appeared to expect criticism from the women they cared for. Whilst the women may be critical about the system of health care and of the quality of the health care they received in this study they were rarely critical of the individuals providing it.

Health professionals would be supported in their work by:

- accurate feedback
- the opportunity to discuss their interventions.

❏ **Organisational issues**

The system of health care provided for women miscarrying early in pregnancy will vary in different locations. In the hospital in this study women are normally admitted to hospital for an ERPC under general anaesthesia. Attention to the following issues would improve women's experiences.

GP care prior to admission to hospital

Apart from the women who had a history of problem pregnancies or were a medical emergency the route to hospital was an obstacle course. The women felt their symptoms were trivialised or were falsely reassured about them by locum GPs. It is essential that the symptoms of miscarriage are taken seriously.

Location of hospital care

However competent the staff, the location in this hospital of women who are miscarrying in the A&E dept and the emergency ward was detrimental to women's care. The pressures of acute emergency work are in conflict with the needs of women who are miscarrying.

Planned care

Unless there is a medical emergency women received better care when they were part of the planned system of care. Women were able to prepare themselves for admission and arrange for their partner, friend or relative to accompany them, time spent 'hanging around' being reduced. When the hospital stay is brief and care compartmentalised, failing to keep to the planned system of care means that women miss out on the help that is available.

Making the opportunity to talk

Health care for women who miscarry is characterised by a chain of care including the GP, the A&E department and the EPAC, the ultrasound department, the emergency ward and theatre, normally within a 24-hour period, during which there is limited contact between health professional and patient. It is easy for women to pass through the system of care without having the opportunity to talk in any depth with a professional about the miscarriage. This could be overcome by:

- providing each woman with a named member of staff who has the responsibility to make him/herself available to talk to the woman if she wishes
- all staff the woman encounters throughout her health care being more prepared to discuss both the physical and emotional aspects of the miscarriage with her, if she wishes, and not assuming that someone else has or will do this.

Discharge procedure

All women must be provided with the opportunity for discussion with an informed member of staff before discharge from hospital. In addition written information must be given to every woman, covering the basic causes of miscarriage, the physical and emotional after-effects, the implications for her partner and family, advice about resuming sexual intercourse, use of tampons and bathing, advice about preconceptual care and trying again, details of relevant local support groups and contact numbers for counselling help.

Follow-up care

The quality of the follow-up care a woman received was dependent on her relationship with and the quality of her GP. The experienced GPs, aware of the limitations of hospital care from the woman's viewpoint, gave importance to their role in follow-up care: medical check, providing information, picking up the pieces, being available, possibly over a period of time. GPs must be more proactive in providing follow-up care, in recognising the physical and emotional consequences of miscarriage and in making provision for non-medical counselling.

■ Suggestions for further reading

Journal of Reproductive and Infant Psychology (1994) **12**(1). Special issue: Understanding the experience and emotional consequences of miscarriage.

Miscarriage Association Newsletter, available from the Miscarriage Association (see Appendix I).

Moulder, C. (1995) *Miscarriage: Women's Experiences and Needs*, London, Pandora Press/HarperCollins.

Oakley, A., McPherson, A. and Roberts, H. (1990) *Miscarriage*, Harmondsworth, Penguin.

Chapter 3

Early termination of pregnancy

■ Introduction

❏ The local health care system for the early termination of pregnancy

The women in this study seeking a termination of pregnancy approached their GP and were referred to a consultant obstetrician and gynaecologist at an outpatient clinic at the local hospital. Once the termination was agreed an appointment was made for the termination at the day surgery unit. The women could themselves have approached a private clinic in the area or been referred by their GP. There is an NHS contract for a charitable organisation to provide NHS-funded care for some local residents. One woman said her GP discussed this option with her but she could see no benefits in going to the clinic. It was assumed for the other women that they would not be able to afford the fee. There are voluntary pregnancy advisory services in the town but none of the women approached these agencies.

When an abnormality is detected early in pregnancy women are offered a termination of the pregnancy. If they wish to go ahead they are normally admitted to the gynaecology ward of the hospital, which offers more privacy and the option of staying overnight.

Counselling is not routinely available. Women can seek counselling help privately but need to have the resources to do this. The GP can refer to the practice counsellor if one is available or alternatively the hospital doctor can refer a woman to the gynaecological social worker, although this would be unusual.

The current system of health care is characterised by what one woman called 'conveyor belt care'. The opportunity for contact between woman and health professional is limited, the hospital stay is short, normally under 12 hours, and follow-up care (unless the termination is for abnormality) is minimal. It is a system in which it is easy not to talk about the termination, the reason for the woman's admission to hospital.

❏ Professionals' attitudes to termination of pregnancy

> On the one hand it is a very serious matter and should be treated as
> such. On the other hand if too much emphasis is put on it, it becomes
> impossible for both women and staff.

This experienced nurse summed up the dilemma for staff providing a termination service as a 'delicate balancing act', a view that was widely
supported. It appears that all staff involved in termination services have to
take into account the social, emotional and physical realities for the women
and themselves.

The nitty gritty of the termination procedure was universally found by
staff to be 'distasteful' (nurse), 'really rather sordid' (consultant) and
'difficult to talk about, unpleasant and distressing' (SHO). Many of the
professionals interviewed described how distressing they had found their
involvement with the termination of pregnancy early in their careers but
how they had learned to 'cope with it' and 'get on with it', although many
acknowledged their intense dislike of seeing the human form.

Professionals' views about whether the termination of pregnancy was
experienced by women as a loss varied from those who thought it a gross
assumption to view termination in this way to those who thought there was
always an element of loss, although women would vary in the extent to
which it was acknowledged. It was recognised that some women coped with
termination by disassociating the notion of pregnancy from what was
happening to them whilst others were less able to do this. The responsibility
for making the decision to bring about the end of the pregnancy and the
guilt that may follow were widely recognised as an additional element in the
experience of termination. Whilst caring for women who had repeated
terminations or those who appeared to be flippant was universally considered frustrating and difficult by GPs, hospital doctors and nurses alike, it
was generally thought that most women did not make the decision lightly.

Understanding the difficult circumstances some women found
themselves in, along with the belief that they were providing a necessary and
high-quality service which is helpful to women, appeared to sustain staff in
doing this difficult job. One SHO summed it up thus:

> I have a strong belief that it is part of the service that should be
> offered; contraception will always fail, some women will always live in
> difficult circumstances and be unable to provide for a child and
> children should be wanted.

In addition the nurses on the unit were helped by the flexible and
supportive working environment where tasks are shared and feelings
discussed. Other staff appeared to have little opportunity to discuss the
issues raised by the termination of pregnancy either informally with
colleagues or more formally as part of their professional development.

Several staff described how their attitudes to the termination of pregnancy had changed over time with the development of personal and professional experience. An experienced nurse, a registrar and an SHO all described how, earlier in their careers, they would not take part in the termination of pregnancy but how their views had changed. Some staff indicated how their personal experience of pregnancy and parenthood had influenced their views.

None of the staff interviewed considered their work with the termination of pregnancy a source of personal distress. They can choose not be involved. One nurse said she did not 'approve' of termination but would never show it and, from the women she looked after who rated her care highly, there is no evidence that she did. Termination was considered a routine part of professionals' work, only the occasional case with particularly difficult circumstances causing them personal concern.

However, there was more general concern among less experienced staff, the junior doctors and some of the nurses on the day surgery unit about how much to say and how to talk to women about termination. For example, one SHO, who felt he could not collude with a woman who was requesting her outpatient appointment be brought forward on the grounds that 'there's nothing really there' and 'it isn't really a baby now', explained that the heart beats from an early gestation but worried that this was the wrong thing to say and had caused the woman additional distress.

❑ The women

Background information

Table 3.1 summarises the background information about the six women recruited to the study. They ranged in age from 21 to 36 years and the gestation of their pregnancy varied from approximately 8 to 14 weeks at the time of the termination. It was anticipated (based on both the GP's and the consultant's assessment) that Debbie was around 11 weeks pregnant and not 14 as was discovered at the termination. All had a suction termination. None had had a termination before. All the women apart from Heather requested a termination of the pregnancy, which was agreed to on the grounds that the continuation of the pregnancy would damage their physical or mental health. Heather's pregnancy was terminated on the grounds of severe fetal abnormality.

Apart from Heather all of the women were in a stable relationship. Ros, who had a child, was more settled in her life whilst the others were experiencing a period of change, rethinking their future or making changes in their work, education or accommodation. Although no very young or older women are included in the study, nor those who have repeat terminations, there is no reason to assume these are not typical of many of the women seeking a termination of pregnancy under the NHS at this local hospital.

Table 3.1 Early termination: background information

	Age (years)	Relationship	Reproductive history	Occupation	Reason for termination
Sally	30	married 18 months	first pregnancy	unemployed; journalist/counsellor	continuation of the pregnancy would damage the woman's physical or mental health
Gina	22	engaged	first pregnancy	temp. work as care assistant; applying for professional courses	as above
Debbie	21	cohab 18 months	second pregnancy; first pregnancy – early miscarriage unconfirmed	care assistant on sick leave due to depression	as above
Hilary	22	cohab 18 months	first pregnancy	unemployed; further education pending	as above
Ros	36	cohab 3 years	second pregnancy; 14-month-old child	part-time book-keeper	as above
Heather	23	single, unstable relationship	first pregnancy	unemployed	severe fetal abnormality

Table 3.2 Early termination: women's experiences of the pregnancy

	Gestation at termination (weeks)	Symptoms of pregnancy experienced	Views about this pregnancy	Thoughts about the pregnancy/baby
Sally	12	physically ill, acute stomach pains, consulted GP	'not the right time, not the right pregnancy'; an illness to be cured; expected to miscarry	at the time: 'some cells that weren't meant to be there'; 6 months later: 'loss of a baby'
Gina	10	none reported	unplanned; an accident	started to think about it as a baby but blocked it out
Debbie	11/14	nausea, aching, food fads, thought symptoms imagined	deeply ambivalent; wants children but knows unable to cope now	thought of it as a baby and felt protective
Hilary	12	nausea and pain, consulted GP because of illness	an illness to be cured	at scan saw 'a dot' on the screen and wished she hadn't because it made her think of a baby
Ros	8	tiredness, nausea, aching, nasty taste in mouth	initially excited then realised inability to cope with a second child; an illness	'an illness'; 'it wasn't anything at that stage, nothing really just a blob'; tried not to think about it
Heather	12	tiredness, aching, food fads	pleased, wanted to be pregnant; concerned she was infertile	excited by seeing baby moving at scan; had collected baby clothes and equipment

Women's response to the pregnancy

Heather had not used contraception for several years and said she had wanted to be pregnant for some time. She had begun to fear she was infertile and had approached her GP for help. None of the other women had planned to be pregnant. Apart from Ros, who had not used contraception because she considered she was at a safe time in her cycle, they reported that they were pregnant as a result of contraceptive failure. The discovery of the pregnancy was a crisis for all of them. They were faced with the decision of whether to continue with the pregnancy and were confronted with their feelings about pregnancy and motherhood as well as the reality of their current life circumstances. Gina, for example, realised that, faced with the prospect of a child, her relationship was not as permanent as she had thought whilst Ros was confronted with her ambivalence about a second child. Table 3.2 summarises the women's experiences of the pregnancy.

The psychological and social impact, along with their experience of the physical symptoms, appears to influence the women's interpretations of the physical reality of the pregnancy. Heather was excited by her pregnancy and by seeing the baby move on the scan. She had started to collect baby equipment and to prepare herself for motherhood. Although the reasons for terminating their pregnancies were different she was not alone in thinking of the pregnancy in terms of a baby. Gina initially thought about the pregnancy as a baby, encouraged by her fiancé's wish to have a child. She read leaflets about maternity care and how to have a healthy pregnancy. Once her decision was made she described herself blocking out the reality of the pregnancy and stopped herself thinking of a baby.

Debbie realised how much she wanted children but knew she could not cope at present. She was depressed and on sick leave from work, concerned about the stability of her relationship and described herself as 'mixed up'. She had sought counselling help in an attempt to resolve some difficult family issues. Debbie clearly thought about her pregnancy in terms of a baby and had made minor changes in her life:

> I did start to do things differently as a sort of protection. I ate corn flakes because it's got folic acid and it's supposed to be preventative for spina bifida and I didn't lift heavy things... because I wasn't sure at the time what I wanted to do about it... I was very careful with what I was doing and sometimes I would lay down at night and sort of hold my stomach and I'd had dreams that I was laying next to my boyfriend saying, 'Don't let them take it away.'

Debbie's confusion shows throughout her account of the termination of her pregnancy. She did not protect herself from the reality of the pregnancy as the other women appeared to do.

Sally and Hilary described and related to their pregnancy as an illness that had to be cured. They initially consulted their GPs because of acute stomach pains and were shocked to discover they were pregnant. Both were seen in the A&E department and scanned to exclude the possibility of ectopic pregnancy. Sally reported that she was told the fetal heart was sluggish and she might miscarry, which confirmed her view that the pregnancy was 'not right':

> It never occurred to me to keep it because of the pain... my instinct all along was that this was not right, my body was rejecting this in some way. There was no question of going through with it but equally there was no question in my mind that I wanted to wait for a miscarriage... I had formed no emotional attachment whatsoever with the contents of my uterus... It wasn't a baby – it was some cells that unfortunately weren't meant to be there and I knew that from the way my body had reacted, not from my mind but from my body... If it had been a normal pregnancy it might have been... a different story.

Experiencing the pregnancy as problematic and as an illness appeared to make the decision easier for Sally. Hilary viewed her pregnancy similarly. Her concern focused on medical aspects of the experience and her anxiety on the general anaesthetic. Ros already had a child and quickly recognised her symptoms for what they were but defined this pregnancy, in contrast to her first, as an illness:

> You don't feel well and I suppose we never really looked at it as a baby... I wasn't feeling too good so it was an illness to be treated... If we really felt deeply about it it would be harder... It's just a blob isn't it? It's nothing, there's nothing there.

Regardless of the women's interpretation of the pregnancy there were clear phases in their experience:

- *realisation of the pregnancy:* recognition of the symptoms or diagnosis by the GP
- *making the decision:* either alone or with her partner, a friend or relative or with professional help (consultant obstetrician or counsellor)
- *arranging the termination:* the GP consultation and outpatient appointment
- *the termination:* admission to day surgery unit or gynaecological ward
- *afterwards:* physical recovery, psychological and social impact.

■ Care before admission

❏ Making the decision

Termination for abnormality: Heather's case

Heather had agreed to the triple test but had a limited understanding of what might be detected. She had been excited by seeing the baby moving on the scan at ten weeks. It was at the second scan that the severe abnormality was detected. Her first indication that something was wrong was when she asked for a picture of the scan but was told she had better wait. She never did get a picture and resented this. A photograph of the scan was the only tangible evidence of the confirmation of the pregnancy and the baby she could have. She was advised by the sonographer that her baby was 'not developing properly' and she needed to see the consultant obstetrician.

Heather described the consultant as extremely 'nice and straightforward' and said he explained that the abnormality was severe and incompatible with life. She was offered a termination of pregnancy and told that if she wanted to avoid an induced labour she must decide quite quickly. She was given a number to telephone should she wish to discuss it further. She describes herself as deciding during the consultation that she would go ahead with the termination but not saying so because she did not wish to leave the hospital in tears. She phoned later to make the arrangements. She consistently described herself as being clear about her decision and not having an alternative. She did not wish to proceed with a pregnancy for her baby to be stillborn or to die shortly after birth.

Heather appeared calm about her decision, leading the consultant at the time and her GP later to conclude that 'it was not a wanted pregnancy'. Although Heather may have had some ambivalence about the pregnancy she was clear that she wanted a baby; indeed by the second interview she was excited at the prospect that she might be pregnant again but was clear that this one was not to be. She saved her distress until she got home.

The consultant was concerned that Heather had to wait to see him with happily pregnant women and thought there should be someone else for her to talk it over with. She was offered a contact number but no counselling help.

Termination for other reasons: 'the hardest part of the experience'

Apart from Debbie the other women were able, within a relatively short period of time, to be clear that they did not wish to be pregnant at this point in their lives and to make the decision to seek a termination of the pregnancy. Sally and Ros shared their decision with their partners whereas Hilary and Gina, who differed with their partners in their views, made their decision independently. Apart from Ros these women talked over their dilemma with a woman they were close to: a relative or friend. Table 3.3

summarises the sources of counselling and lay support available to the women prior to the termination.

Table 3.3 Early termination: counselling and sources of lay support prior to termination

	Counselling offered by GP	Counselling received	Lay sources of support in decision making
Sally	none	none	husband (a joint decision); mother; girlfriend
Gina	none	none	mother; friend; partner (wished her to continue with pregnancy)
Debbie	none offered because the GP thought she was clear in her decision and she was already seeing the practice counsellor	partner's mother arranged and paid for session with private counsellor	partner (wished her to have a termination); partner's mother
Hilary	GP found telephone number of pregnancy helpline in the *Yellow Pages*	none	partner who accepted her decision despite wishing to continue with pregnancy; mother, cousin
Ros	none offered; GP could have referred to practice counsellor but did not because she seemed clear in her decision	none	partner (joint decision)
Heather	no contact with GP	none	mother

These were private decisions. The women did not seek professional help at the decision-making stage and were not well informed about sources of counselling help had they wanted it. Sally would have welcomed the opportunity to talk over her decision with a skilled outsider but did not do so. Ros and Hilary did not wish to discuss their decision with anyone else.

Debbie was confused about what to do and was eventually helped by discussing her situation with a counsellor, as she describes:

> From day to day I still had doubts... shall I, shan't I? One day I'd think, 'Yes it's the best thing to do' and I could see myself in the summer being able to wear a bikini and do all the things that I would normally do. Go back to college like I wanted... Another day I would see myself... pregnant and bringing up a baby... It was like that from day to day until I saw that woman... She'd actually been through a termination and she'd actually been through bringing up a baby without a stable relationship as well. To be able to talk to someone that had been through both. That is what really made my mind up.

Debbie saw a counsellor at a voluntary organisation, arranged and paid for by her boyfriend's mother; she would not have had the resources to organise this on her own. Although she was intermittently seeing the male counsellor at her GP practice she did not feel she could discuss this decision with a man.

❏ The GP appointment

Heather did not see her GP prior to the termination. Once their pregnancy was confirmed all the women approached their GP to request a referral for its termination. Only Debbie made the appointment with her GP to seek advice or help with the decision. They all expected to have to justify their decision and that obstacles would be put in their way. They invariably approached a GP with whom they had little previous contact. Table 3.4 summarises the women's and GP's views of the consultation prior to the termination.

The GPs were concerned to safeguard their patient's health and well-being, whether by ruling out the possibility of ectopic pregnancy or by ascertaining that the woman was sure she had made the decision right for her and was not under pressure from her partner or family. Both the women and the GPs described the appointment as focused on confirming the pregnancy and gestation, establishing that the woman was clear about her decision, explaining the options and giving information, although the effects of the pressures of the lack of time, the sensitivity of termination and the potentially different agendas of doctor and patient may work against this being achieved.

The women's evaluation of their GP care varied (Table 3.5). Sally and Gina were surprised by the brevity of the appointment with the GP and the lack of discussion about their reasons for seeking the termination, being critical of the off-hand manner in which they considered they had been treated. They described referral to the consultant as automatic. Gina, who said her appointment with the locum GP had lasted three minutes, was reluctant to discuss her situation:

> Her [the GP's] immediate reaction was asking if it was my first child...
> So it made it quite difficult for me to turn round and say, 'Actually I don't want to keep it'... and she said to me, 'What does the father think?' I said he supports me. I didn't want to go into it... I didn't know her from anyone else... I felt she was looking at me, criticising my decision because she asked if I were engaged. Fine, that was it...
> No-one else said anything else to me at all.

In order to speed up the outpatient referral Gina and her mother subsequently approached another GP in the practice who was more familiar to them.

Table 3.4 Early termination: GP care prior to termination

	Purpose of GP consultation from woman's point of view	Women's views of GP consultation	GPs' views
Sally	to diagnose illness and provide treatment; to arrange termination	over time saw three different GPs; lack of continuity, time and discussion unhelpful	lack of continuity a problem; accurate diagnosis of potential ectopic pregnancy rather than feelings about a problem pregnancy was main concern
Gina	to gain agreement for termination	three minute appointment with locum GP, who appeared disapproving and was ignorant of the local service; resented question about the father's view and lack of discussion; later spoke to family GP who was helpful	family GP assessed that she was very sure about her decision and had mother's support
Debbie	to share her dilemma, discuss options, gain information	saw GP jointly with her partner; GP mistakenly congratulated her on pregnancy; GP understanding and non-judgemental; lack of discussion and explanation of medical and bureaucratic procedure	a brave and articulate young woman who had made a difficult decision; knew of personal circumstances making motherhood very difficult; insufficient time
Hilary	to diagnose illness and provide treatment; to arrange termination	valued non-judgemental brief discussion about 'how pregnancy would fit in with things'; telephone number given of voluntary pregnancy advice service	assessed that Hilary was clear in her own mind, decision being made before appointment; insufficient time
Ros	to gain agreement for termination	chose to see GP she did not know; GP asked lots of questions, which was necessary but distressing because it made the pregnancy real	thought that Ros was quite clear what she wanted
Heather	no consultation	—	—

Table 3.5   Early termination: women's perceptions of care

	GP care	Outpatient appointment	Inpatient care	Place cared for in hospital
Sally	4	2	1	day surgery unit
Gina	4	2	1	day surgery unit
Debbie	4	4	2	day surgery unit
Hilary	1	1	1	day surgery unit
Ros	1	1	1	day surgery unit
Heather	1	1	2	gynaecology ward

1 = very helpful
2 = helpful
3 = neither helpful nor unhelpful
4 = unhelpful
5 = very unhelpful

Although Debbie had a longer consultation with her GP she was critical of the inadequate information she was given and the lack of opportunity for discussion. Debbie probably appeared more decisive than she felt. She made a direct request for a termination when she was very confused about continuing with the pregnancy. The GP knew of her difficult circumstances and thought Debbie was making a hard but sensible decision. However, Debbie valued the GP's accepting approach, as she describes:

> She was caring and understanding. I could see that in her eyes and face. I do think she didn't think badly of me.

Ros and Hilary also appreciated the understanding, non-judgemental approach of their GPs, whom they felt were concerned about their welfare. The GPs stressed that their role was to help the women to think through the issues:

> A lot of what we're trying to achieve is to try and take responsibility for themselves and to make their own decisions about what is right for them... I would not try to push what I might think... One has to try and let them put the possible problems that they may come across to them and say, 'Have you thought about this? Have you thought about that?'

Ros felt her GP respected her. She described his asking routine questions and checking with her that it was what she really wanted. Whilst she thought this was important she found it distressing as it gave the pregnancy a reality it had not had before. She describes the dilemma:

In some ways you want people to be concerned about you but on the other hand it's just more distressing... It would have been harder had he [GP] put more obstacles in my way... They are not there to sit in judgement, they are there to offer a service... Although it would have been nice to have had someone care, I think the way they handled it is probably better because it is not as distressing.

The GP appointment provided limited opportunity for some of the women to talk through the medical consequences but not the personal implications of the decision they were making. Hilary's GP gave her the telephone number of a pregnancy advice service in case she wished to talk over her decision. He was concerned not to give her the number of an organisation with strong moral views and looked in the *Yellow Pages* for the appropriate telephone number. Both Ros's and Debbie's GP assumed that they did not need further counselling help so did not refer them to the practice counsellor (see Table 3.3 above). Several GPs expected that the outpatient appointment would provide an opportunity for a more extensive discussion.

❑ **The outpatient appointment**

Women's experiences

The biggest thing is the expectation of being told off... For a woman to actually get to a gynae clinic to request termination she's had to go through so many different barriers; ...deciding with her husband or partner what they're going to do, the personal decision; they've got to go to the GP, they've got to explain the reasons; they've got to be referred on... All along the line the majority of them feel very embarrassed, they feel guilty and they are scared that someone is going to say 'No' or 'You're stupid' and 'Why have you done that?'

Consultant

This consultant was correct in his view that women experience arranging a termination as a series of hurdles to be overcome and expect to be judged. Indeed, all of the women thought the outpatient appointment would be difficult and that they would have to justify their decision. Apart from Debbie and Hilary, who both expected they would be admitted for the termination that day, the criticisms they had were relatively minor: that they were passed from pillar to post, there was lots of hanging around and it was bureaucratic.

Contrary to their expectations the women found the outpatient appointment more relaxed than they anticipated, as Ros describes:

You go along there thinking they're going to give you a hard time and make it even harder for you. But they were straightforward medical questions and... the nurse was very good and very considerate towards me... She didn't actually say anything about what you were having done but she was very considerate... you don't really want anyone to sit in judgement because it is a hard decision to come to... you don't really want anyone to challenge you... I was dreading most going for this consultation because I just didn't know what they were going to say to me.

They all described the nursing and medical staff as sympathetic, kind and concerned. Accounts from both the women and the doctors confirm that the consultation consisted of an examination to confirm the gestation and practical information about the nature of surgery, the possible side-effects and the physical after-effects. For Gina it was surprisingly routine and for Ros a bit like an ordinary antenatal appointment. The women expected that they would have to discuss their reasons for requesting a termination; some women had been prepared for this by their GP and were surprised to discover not only that there was little opportunity for this but also that it was not deemed important.

Medical views

It is clearly assumed by the medical staff that, by the time a woman reaches the outpatient department, she is clear about her decision. As one consultant said, 'I don't think they want any questioning. They've been through all that.' Broadly speaking, they subscribed to the view that a woman must be the one to make her decision and the role of the medical profession is to support her in her choice. The hospital doctors (consultants, registrars and SHOs) were unanimous in their view that it was neither possible, owing to the pressure of time and their lack of counselling skills, nor their role at an outpatient appointment to discuss at length feelings about the termination or the reason for it, as one consultant describes:

I tend to assume that by the time they have got to me they are certain... The GP often puts in the letter if there is any hesitation. I always say to them... 'I'm sorry that you're here and I'm sorry that this has happened. Are you absolutely sure that... you want a termination?'... You can go into it a bit more if you pick up at that stage that there is a problem. And there is no way in a busy gynae clinic that I can do any more than that. You don't have any counselling services available... If she hides that there is a problem I wouldn't find it.

An SHO echoed this view but pointed out that if a woman was requesting repeat abortions or if she appeared very unsure he would challenge her. One registrar stressed that in reality, beyond a few questions, there is not enough time for discussion in any detail. Another said he only intervened if the woman appeared unsure, when he would suggest she go away and think about it. He thought asking a woman to justify herself unnecessary and a potential source of additional distress, but appreciated this was not what women expected:

> Women often come in expecting confrontation and having to justify themselves and you can tell that because of their surprise when you... start taking their history, like not making a big thing about it because it isn't a big thing. If we as practitioners don't approve of termination we don't have to be there. So it's not our place to judge.

There are clearly different expectations of the outpatient appointment. Table 3.6 summarises the different views. The GPs on the whole expected a more lengthy consultation. The hospital doctors took the view that discussion about the reason for the termination and the woman's feelings about it was the responsibility of the GP. The women excepted to be given 'a hard time' and to be 'judged'.

❑ The implications of the present system of care

It is easy to see how Debbie ended up feeling she had not talked properly to anybody:

> The whole thing all the way through seemed to be rushed through with no discussion... it was booked, it was done and that was it. Everybody was very kind but... everything was very brief and it was as if they didn't want to talk to you about it too much because they didn't want to bring up any problems or upset you or... it was all sort of rushed through.

Several of the women echoed Debbie's feeling that nobody wanted to talk about it and contrasted the personal and medical significance of the event. Ros had a sense of 'unreality' about the termination because it was all so unspoken. Hilary was surprised at 'the general ease of everything'.

These women were surprised that they were not questioned more extensively and assumed that they had to present a coping front in order to gain agreement to the termination. They were critical that there was little or no opportunity for discussion throughout the process. However, their views on the need to talk about it differed and, when opportunities did arise, they made limited use of them. Ros, for example, felt it was not necessarily a bad thing that no-one really talks to you: 'you want someone to acknowledge your dilemma and indecision but you don't because that makes it more difficult'. She described her care as 'effective and unintrusive, a background to a difficult and intensely personal decision'.

In addition they feared judgement from the professionals they depended on although there is no evidence from this study that professionals judged

Table 3.6 Early termination: the outpatient appointment

	GPs' expectations	Women's views	Dr seen at outpatient appointment	Hospital doctor's views
Sally	depends who you see as to the service you get; private clinic offers superior care	clear explanation; procedure straightforward	consultant	lack time; assume decision made
Gina	outpatient appointment will involve discussion with consultant	expected to justify her decision; wanted but didn't get explanation for pregnancy whilst on the Pill; an obstacle course; very routine	consultant	assumes GP has discussed decision fully; gives practical information
Debbie	counselling at the hospital is inadequate	thought operation would be done then; an obstacle course; no opportunity for discussion	consultant	lack time; assume decision made
Hilary	women have to justify themselves to the consultant	unsure if operation would be done then; could have asked anything but didn't	consultant (at her request)	only counsel if women unsure; women expect confrontation and do not get it
Ros	full discussion with the consultant offers a 'second bite of the cherry'	expected to be given a hard time; lots of hanging around; very routine and straightforward; no explanation of the procedure	SHO	discussion is GP's role
Heather	–	clear explanation of abnormality, the scan and discussion; questions answered and advice given; offered further telephone contact; very helpful	consultant	best service that could be provided in the circumstances; should not have to wait after scan in antenatal; someone else should be available to see her for further discussion.

these women harshly. Their fears possibly stem from the judgements the women were making about their own actions, which they projected on to those around them.

The system of health care as it operates locally at present within the current legislative framework does not help women to discuss their decision or their feelings about it should they need or wish to. The professionals they encounter are responsible for approving their request for a termination. No opportunity is routinely offered for women to discuss impartially the implications of their decision.

■ Inpatient care

❏ The day surgery unit and gynaecology ward

Women undergoing termination of pregnancy are normally admitted to the day surgery unit at the local hospital unless there are special circumstances and they need longer-term care, in which case they are admitted to the gynaecological ward. Termination of pregnancy is only a part of the work of the day surgery unit, although of late an increasing part. Staff on the unit recognise the problems of 'mixed lists' and the tensions that can arise when caring for women undergoing a termination of pregnancy at the same time as caring for those with fertility problems. Although in general terms both the women and staff described the facilities provided in the unit as satisfactory, the general lack of privacy was criticised. The provision of a room where staff could talk with a woman confidentially and of shower and bidet facilities would be welcomed.

At the time of the study the nursing staff on the day surgery unit formed a stable and mature group, most of whom had worked together for several years. The work rota for the unit is organised on a flexible basis, enabling the nursing staff to move between the ward, theatre and recovery on a session basis if they wish. All the nursing staff interviewed in the day surgery unit said they felt part of a close and supportive team, comprising the nursing staff. Openness in talking about difficult cases and about issues as they arose was particularly valued, as was being able to swap tasks according to individual skills. One nurse described how difficult she found it to talk to women about their feelings, so she would find a colleague who was more skilled to do this. There was a monthly meeting, which was described as useful: 'you can bring anything up'. The support identified by the staff was mainly informal and a function of the good working relationships between the nursing staff and with the sister in charge, who was approachable and whose professional skills and leadership were valued.

The gynaecology ward has recently been refurbished and offers improved facilities. The nursing staff described a supportive and well-run ward. They care for a patient undergoing termination of pregnancy about once a week and occasionally for miscarriage patients. Women who have an ectopic pregnancy are transferred here from the emergency ward following surgery. There is not such a high turnover of patients on this ward and staff take a pride in individualising care.

❑ Women's views of inpatient care

> The other doctors I've seen (apart from my GP) have been wonderful and the nursing staff were tremendously helpful. They offered all the advice. There was no feeling at any point that I was doing anything wrong. There was no sort of feeling of being morally judged, which was a huge relief. Sally

All the women considered they had received good inpatient care (see Table 3.5 above). The staff, both nursing and medical (anaesthetists as well as gynaecologists), were all described as non-judgemental, kind, sensitive and appropriate. The women felt well cared for, even though in Hilary's words it was 'conveyor belt care'. They described the termination as viewed as a minor operation, routine and straightforward, an approach they found helpful. They experienced the staff as non-intrusive, the nurses as 'really, really nice' and available to answer questions, although they did not ask many. They were generally unprepared for the procedure they were about to undergo, perhaps a function of their anxiety at their medical appointments prior to admission. Gina and Hilary, who were anxious about the anaesthetic, were reassured by the anaesthetists. Heather, who was similarly anxious, was extremely well cared for on a side room of the gynaecological ward.

Two particular aspects of their experience stand out in the women's accounts of their inpatient care; firstly, the significance of the admission procedure, and secondly the lack of explicit discussion about the termination, the reason for their admission.

❑ Admission

Arriving at the hospital and waiting to be admitted was an anxious time for all the women. Debbie was aware that she could still change her mind. Ros described a sense of personal shame, how she felt a bit 'unclean' and questioned what she was doing. Like all the women she compared herself with the others waiting to be admitted, noting their age, whether they were alone or with a partner or friend and whether they appeared upset and made incorrect assumptions about why they were there:

> I felt I was the only one in for a termination... Sitting around in the waiting room, I suppose wondering what other people are in for. Then you're sort of called in one at a time... the receptionist doesn't give you any idea of what is happening, just take a seat and you are

waiting for someone to call your name. As I was the last in line, everyone else had been in, had been briefed, they did come along and ask the normal questions and gave you an idea of what time the operation would be, asking do you wear jewellery, nail varnish, I don't know quite why, they're just sort of normal operation questions...

The women are acutely sensitive to the way the staff respond to them and can easily misinterpret what is said. When the nurse asked if her mother would be at home to look after her afterwards Debbie, who has a difficult and unhappy relationship with her mother, felt it was assumed that she was too young to be living with her boyfriend and sad her mother could not be there for her.

Heather appreciated being greeted by name. Recognising her anxiety the nurse allocated to her spent a lot of time with her, shared her own experience of a termination and arranged for a friend to visit. The nurse underestimated her importance to Heather.

In contrast to the women's anxieties the admission process was very matter-of-fact and routine. However, from the woman's point of view the admission nurse played an important role in putting her at ease, preparing her and creating the opportunity for questions to be asked. One of the nurses described her role:

almost like a mum... for some of the younger ones because they need someone to be able to relate to, to ask the questions they couldn't ask other people... If they are emotional we don't actually counsel them as such, we do have to listen to what they are saying, perhaps advise them and comfort them.

The admission nurse was one of the few professionals throughout the whole process of the termination with whom the women had any opportunity to establish contact. All the women in the study chose the nurse who admitted them as one of the health professionals significant in their care.

❑ Talking about the termination

The absence of frank discussion about the termination was a theme that recurred for some of the women throughout their health care but the women's need for information, explanation, the opportunity to talk about the termination or just the acknowledgement that it had happened varied. Talking about the termination was clearly an issue for some of the nursing staff as well, as one of the nurses describes:

I feel really inadequate and I don't want to say the wrong things to them and I don't want them to feel worse then they already do... But I feel that they feel that they can't open up to you because they see how busy it is, they see how rushed it is and even if they do they always say I'm sorry for taking up so much of your time. And I think 'God that's why I'm here.' But I don't feel equipped anyway really.

The nurses varied in experience, particularly in how confident they felt about talking with women. Most of the nurses were realistic about the lack of opportunity for women to talk over their feelings either before or after the termination. Concerns about how to approach women and how much encouragement to give women to talk were common, along with fears that they 'would put their foot in it' or would 'undo things already done' – a woman might want to change her mind when this was clearly impossible. The less experienced nurses felt less able to talk to women, particularly if they were overtly distressed, one describing how she always found a more skilled member of staff to talk to women if necessary.

Heather felt adequately prepared for the operation and had few questions but the reasons for the termination were not discussed. The nurses on the ward were initially unaware of the abnormality as her maternity notes were unavailable, so the issue was not addressed. This was not significant for Heather.

Sally and Gina, both of whom had a general interest in women's health issues and detailed knowledge about abortion prior to their own experience, felt informed about procedures on their admission to hospital. They had few questions to ask but were both confident that the staff caring for them would answer any queries they had. Gina emphasised how the nurses made themselves available although she had little she wanted to ask. Sally describes the nurse who admitted her:

She had some spunk about her. I liked her. She had her feet firmly on the ground, made me feel very safe, as if I'd get no crap out of her at all. She would tell me what was what.

Debbie, Hilary and Ros, who did not have this background knowledge, felt ignorant of the process and unprepared for what they were to go through. Information that had been made available to them at an earlier stage in their health care was insufficient. Although the staff were consistently described as caring and approachable these women did not feel able to ask questions about the termination. Ros found it impossible to talk about something so personal in such a public place. Hilary described herself as an assertive person but in hospital found it impossible to ask even basic questions about what she should do and what was going to happen. Debbie describes her own feelings about this:

Nobody explained to me what was going to happen to me. You had the leaflets telling you about it and I'd read it so I knew and I'd asked my mum... It just seemed that nobody wanted to talk about it, nobody wanted to speak about it... I mean what's the anaesthetic like?

What do they do in the operating theatre? You know explain it to me properly... I thought they would say to me, 'Well haven't you read it? It's on the bit of paper you've been given.' ...I don't know. I felt like I couldn't ask... It would have been nice if the doctor had said to me in the first place, 'Would you like me to explain the procedure from here onwards?' ...If I wanted to know I could have said yes and if I wanted to block it out then I would say, 'I'd rather not know.'

It was not only the lack of specific information that worried Ros but also the lack of acknowledgement of the reality of the event, which she thought was due to the complex nature of termination and the moral dilemmas posed. She describes the doctor coming to see her afterwards:

I know the girl next to me... whatever she was having done they discussed it more or less but when he came to me he said, 'everything's OK'... He didn't say exactly what it really was as if... it's unspoken.

The unspoken nature of the event made it seem unreal, leaving her feeling as if the termination had never happened, a feeling that lasted for some time after her discharge from hospital. However, on reflection, she thought the lack of discussion was a good thing as it made it less overtly distressing.

That it is clearly appropriate for some if not all women that the event remains unacknowledged and undefined presents staff caring for women with a series of dilemmas. Women have to indicate clearly that they want information or need to talk, which, as indicated above, they are not always able to do. The nursing staff were clearly sensitive to individual need. Their ideas about good care focused on 'conveying a feeling of understanding' and 'honest explanation', excellent medical care being taken for granted.

❑ Disposal

A sensitive issue

The handling and disposal of the products of pregnancy is an unpleasant aspect of the termination of pregnancy but if the operation is viewed as a straightforward, minor medical intervention and nothing to do with a pregnancy or baby it is unlikely to be viewed as a complex issue. Personal reactions of the staff caring for these women varied from those of the SHO, for whom it was just not an issue, and the nurse, who did not find the process of the operation difficult or offensive, to those of an SEN who found it much harder, as she describes:

when you've got to remove the little sac from the tube... and you've got to empty that bit and put it in the box. I find that really hard to do... especially if it's a pregnancy that's gone on... I try and find myself busy in the recovery room.

For her it did not get easier with increased experience or age. She was acutely aware that her own successful pregnancies and miscarriage made it harder. Another experienced nurse thought everybody hated disposal but that some people found it more distressing than others. She said she hated it, got particularly distressed if she saw the human form and admitted she tried not to look. She was adamant that she never wanted to get used to it.

Health professionals' views on the system of disposal

Aborted material from suction termination of pregnancy is strained to reduce the liquid and collected together in a 'Sharps' box. It is sealed and transported to another hospital site, where it is incinerated. Unlike the products of conception following a miscarriage there is no individual packaging of waste material. This system of disposal is widely considered by staff to be an improvement on the previous system of using the sluice. However, some of the nursing staff were unclear why the system had changed and unsure of what happened after the box left the unit. For a couple of nurses their lack of knowledge appeared to fuel fears that the material may be used for experimentation which was considered inappropriate.

Some staff clearly felt there was still scope for improving the system. One senior nurse thought the aborted material should be packaged separately as a mark of respect. Another nurse thought this a good idea if it meant you did not have to look. However, many staff taking a more pragmatic view – 'What difference does it really make?' thought the present system acceptable and would concur with the views of one of the consultants who considered separate incineration unnecessary:

It think that's a bit silly... It's window dressing. I don't know who it's to make feel better... If a patient feels strongly about disposal they will allow them to make their own arrangements. It's not our property, it's theirs.

Aside from the consultants and most of the nursing staff directly involved with the procedure there is considerable ignorance about disposal arrangements. The nurses on the gynaecological ward and many of the junior hospital doctors, including registrars, said they did not know what happened, some not having thought about it until asked for the purposes of this research. Likewise many of the GPs, who may be the person a woman turns to after the event, were unaware of what was involved. Without full knowledge of the system for disposal no professional can answer a woman's questions or discuss the issue easily with her.

Talking with women about disposal

Disposal was not an issue for all the women in the study. Heather was unaware and did not want to know what had happened to the remains of her pregnancy. Gina and Hilary said they did not think about it and Ros clearly defined her pregnancy as 'nothing', so disposal was not a cause for concern. Sally, owing to her previous employment, had accurate, detailed information about disposal methods so had no need for further information. Debbie, who was critical about the lack of explicit information about the procedure, did not have this information, and what happened to the baby remained an unanswered question. One month after the termination she wrote, 'I often wonder where the baby went, what they do with it', a concern she echoed two months later.

Although a few staff said they would fudge the issue or tell white lies to make the information they gave more acceptable most thought that if women wanted information it should be communicated honestly to them. However, the onus is clearly on women to broach the subject. All of the doctors interviewed (gynaecologists and GPs) thought it unusual for a woman to want this information following a termination. Some made the assumption that women who choose to have a termination do not think of their pregnancy in terms of a baby and disposal is therefore not an issue. That making a choice to terminate a pregnancy inevitably involves a woman's forfeiting her rights over the fetus may underlie this view. Few had much experience of being asked although one consultant pointed out that ideas about these things were changing and, making the comparison with early miscarriage, thought that more women were likely to ask as it became acceptable to do so.

Questions about disposal were unusual for the nurses as well and often dreaded. Based on her wide experience one of the staff nurses thought that only a few women wanted this information. It was her policy to give general information unless direct questions were asked. She highlights the difficulty in choosing the words to use as well as her own discomfort with the reality of disposal:

> If they want to know what happens, then we will tell them what happens. They don't always understand, and they don't always want to know... You get people who... say, 'Well what happens to the baby?' It's very difficult to explain that with suction you don't actually see anything. And they want to know the sex sometimes and of course... you don't know anything like that at all. How it's going to be disposed of, not many times, but people do ask. And you have to answer truthfully to the best of your ability... I just say that what happens is suction and it goes into a special container and then it is taken away to be disposed of as human tissue... It's very difficult but that's what I say. And then they don't sort of ask any more... I've never had it happen to me that people have said, 'Is it going to be

buried or something?' It's very difficult to say that it is going to be incinerated. I just say it's going to be disposed of.

This nurse had worked out her own way of handling the issue with women. Her experience and comfortable manner may have made it easier for women to approach her.

❑ Postoperative care and discharge from hospital

The women on the day surgery unit all felt well cared for after the operation. They wanted their privacy and to sleep but felt staff were available if needed. Heather was more demanding of attention and, although it was objectively good, was critical of her postoperative care. Her nurse thought she was sensitively keeping an eye on her and checking her bleeding whilst Heather misinterpreted her discretion as inaction.

As long as they are fit and provided there is someone at home to care for them the women were discharged from hospital a few hours after the termination. Only Debbie stayed longer. Her pregnancy was more advanced than initially thought and the procedure therefore more complex. It was suggested she should stay in hospital overnight but she refused.

On discharge from hospital, a process described by one of the nurses as 'goodbye and good luck', a nurse will talk to a woman, providing the opportunity to ask questions. An information sheet is given with general advice about the probable physical and emotional reactions and instructions to consult the hospital or GP if adverse symptoms are experienced. Several of the nurses on the gynaecological and day surgery wards commented on the lack of counselling facilities for women undergoing termination of pregnancy.

Sally and Gina had no queries, felt they knew all they needed to and described the discharge process as straightforward. Hilary, Debbie and Ros all thought that the information they were given was inadequate and felt ill prepared for the way in which their body would react following the termination. Heather similarly felt let down by the informality of the discharge procedure and was unsure what to expect in terms of postoperative bleeding.

■ After discharge from hospital

❑ Health care after the termination

Table 3.7 summarises the women's experiences of health care after the termination. Heather, whose pregnancy was terminated because of an abnormality, was routinely offered follow-up care whilst the other women had to ask for any help they needed. In addition to the support offered by her GP Heather saw the consultant obstetrician and gynaecologist to discuss

Table 3.7 Early termination: health care post-termination

	Health care after termination	Women's views
Sally	GP contraceptive advice; termination not mentioned	would have liked: six week check with GP to be offered routinely, acknowledgement of termination, opportunity to talk over the experience
Gina	not known; planned to contact family planning clinic for contraceptive advice	not known
Debbie	GP for post-termination symptoms of heavy bleeding; re-admission to hospital necessary due to infection; continued with counselling help through GP practice	would have liked easier access to GP; counselling invaluable
Hilary	rang hospital due to concern about post-termination bleeding; GP for contraceptive advice, termination not mentioned	would have liked discussion about when to expect next period, symptoms post-termination and GP to acknowledge termination
Ros	GP for contraceptive advice and problems with lack of menstruation	would have liked discussion with medical person about physical consequences of termination, i.e. bodily changes, when periods should resume, etc.
Heather	follow-up appointment with consultant to discuss abnormality; check-up and discussion with GP prompted by her concern about bleeding	both extremely helpful

the abnormality and future pregnancies. She valued his clear explanation and felt able to ask questions.

The women in general were concerned about the normality of the physical symptoms they were experiencing. Hilary rang the day surgery unit for advice when bleeding started again a few days after her discharge. Debbie, who started to bleed heavily, eventually contacted her GP and was re-admitted to hospital for an ERPC. Apart from specific problems the women said they did not know what changes in their body to expect or when their periods would recommence. They would have welcomed the opportunity to talk over these issues with an experienced professional. Gina continued to be concerned about why she had got pregnant whilst taking the Pill, a question she thought someone would have answered for her by now.

The women also needed contraceptive advice and approached their GP for this. For Ros and Sally contraception had been particularly problematic and resolving these difficulties, which took several months, was a turning point in their recovery. When Sally and Hilary approached their GP for contraception the termination was not mentioned, which they found surprising. Sally felt that the lack of acknowledgement belittled her experience:

It was all family planning related and a follow-up smear and not one of them asked me about the operation. There was no opportunity to talk or any counselling offered or anything like that... It can be so easily trivialised... 'Oh you're going to have a minor op, off you go' and 'You'll be fine. You can have other babies later on.' I mean it's not that simple and a lot of doctors seem to treat it like that.

Debbie continued to meet regularly with the counsellor she had been seeing before she got pregnant. She described the counselling as invaluable in helping her sort out the problems she was experiencing, which had been exacerbated by her pregnancy. None of the other women sought counselling help and none said they wanted it.

❏ Women's reactions in the six months after the termination

Table 3.8 summarises the women's reactions to the termination of their pregnancy at different points in time. It should be noted that Gina and Debbie did not complete the second interview although Debbie completed the diary sheets and spoke on the telephone.

After the termination none of these women expressed any regret at the decision they had made and they were relieved they had got through the experience. Their overwhelming wish was to 'get back to normal' and to 'put the experience behind them' and were determined to do so. Hilary read that she might be depressed, a suggestion she resented:

I just didn't want to be depressed... I'd been feeling really ill and I just thought once it's over and done with... I just want to get back to

Table 3.8 Early termination: women's reactions

	At the time	In the intervening months	Six months after termination	Overall themes in the experience of the pregnancy and termination
Sally	straightforward relief of physical symptoms	one month later described an overwhelming sense of loss; sorting out contraception that suited her was a turning point	no regrets; 'it's well and truly over'; refers to the termination as the 'loss of the baby'	'a small loss' compared with other losses she has had; brought a lot of things into focus, made decisions about the future
Gina	relief	not known	not known	questioned the permanence of the relationship with her partner
Debbie	upset, lonely, thinking how different things could be; rows with boyfriend; determined to make good use of her time	thoughts about the termination lessening over time; physical recovery a turning point	regrets the necessity but knows it was for the best; thinks what the baby would have been like	hardest decision she has ever made; surprised at her inner strength; confronted her with her ideals of parenthood; one more major thing to deal with
Hilary	relief of physical symptoms and illness	'happy and healthy'; surprised how good she felt and how quickly	extremely well physically and emotionally; confident made the right decision	being on her own
Ros	felt ill; had second thoughts in hospital; worried how she would live with it	sorting out irregular periods and contraception was a turning point; relieved not pregnant	no regrets, relief; 'something that happened to me in the past'; glad she does not have another child	resolved couple's differences about having a second child
Heather	upset, but clear about the decision as abnormality incompatible with life	distressed and crying on return home; felt bleak for a couple of days and then 'got on with things'	no regrets, hoping she may be pregnant again	she is not infertile, wants a healthy baby; 'one of the many hard things that have happened'

normal... I don't feel depressed, I haven't got any major regrets, I haven't got any worries... I think for a couple of days I was maybe a little bit tearful... a little bit vulnerable to maybe harsh words spoken... maybe it was just because I was tired and the anaesthetic or whatever. But I haven't been feeling depressed, if anything I am just so relieved to be feeling a little bit better again and knowing that actually now I can start getting on with things again.

Six months later they were surprised how well they felt, saw the termination as part of their history and were getting on with their lives. Only Sally reported a change in the way she thought about the termination. What had been a straightforward medical event had become the loss of her baby, for which she was unprepared. A month after the termination she wrote:

The phrase 'I lost my baby last week' kept going through my mind, even though I hadn't associated the pregnancy with 'a baby' at the time. I somehow felt the need for sympathy and yet didn't feel deserving of it. This conflict was confusing... that week I lost my appetite, I felt isolated and also overwhelmingly tired.

Debbie had been distressed by the termination of her pregnancy but shortly afterwards she was positive about the future:

I feel I need to try and get on with my life and replace... instead of the fact that I haven't had the baby, to replace it and do something good in the year instead... I'm going back to college and I've got to start going back to work soon... I don't actually feel like I want to talk deeply about it and get upset about it at the moment. I don't know whether that will happen later or not but at the moment I seem to have managed to close the door on it and be quite strong.

The misery of the termination was intensified for her by the necessity of re-admission to hospital for an ERPC. She felt she was able to get on with her life once she was physically better. She continued to think about the loss of her baby after the termination but this lessened over time. She did return to work and was hopeful of gaining admission to college.

These women appeared to have incorporated the termination of their pregnancy into the fabric of their lives although they were aware that feelings about the termination may surface again later. There is no evidence from the information gained in the six months of the study to suggest that they were damaged psychologically by the experience. However, the termination had clearly been an event of some significance to them. Gina questioned the permanence of her relationship with her fiancé and, at the time of the first interview, the relationship appeared to be breaking down. Sally made major decisions about giving up her job and plans for her future. Debbie was confronted with her complex feelings about motherhood but had been surprised by her inner strength. For Ros it resolved her dilemmas about having a second child.

■ Conclusion: the ethos of the system of care

There are differences in the system of care for women whose pregnancies are terminated in the first trimester because of an abnormality compared with those whose pregnancies are terminated for other reasons. The former reach hospital by a different route, are cared for in a different location where it is easier to offer more individualised care and follow-up care is routinely offered, whereas this is not the case for the latter. Despite the differences in the way the health care is organised many of the issues for the women remain the same.

The ethos of this system of care is one of respectful caution. There is clearly a delicate balance between on the one hand intrusive questions or disrespect for a private decision and on the other hand neglect, the failure to show genuine concern and offer effective help at a time of personal crisis. This dilemma is apparent throughout the provision of health care for the early termination of pregnancy. It seems it is resolved by professionals erring on the side of caution, making assumptions that women are clear in their minds and will ask for help if they need it.

There appear to be three principles which underpin the provision of the service:

- *acceptance of the woman's decision:* few questions are asked for fear of intruding on an individual's privacy or being seen as moralising
- *Minor medical intervention:* the procedure of the termination is viewed as a minor medical intervention and not necessarily to do with pregnancy
- *Self-responsibility:* women must take responsibility for the decision they have made and ultimately for their own welfare.

A system of this kind demands certain characteristics of women, namely that they are resourceful and psychologically straightforward. It works particularly well for women who are clear about their decision, cope by detaching themselves from the idea of a pregnancy, wish to know little of the procedures involved and have resources beyond the health care system if they need further support. Clearly, not all women can conform to these rather stringent requirements.

■ Issues in good practice arising from the research

❑ Staffing and training

Talking about termination

The women were surprised by the current system of health care, which minimises the significance of the termination and does not facilitate discussion about the personal implications of their decision. However, their need to talk about their decision differed and they made little use of opportunities when they did arise. Health professionals, in respecting a woman's privacy, err on the side of caution in talking about termination. Knowing how much to talk to women and what to say was a concern for some staff, particularly the junior doctors and some of the nursing staff. Yet it is hard for women to ask questions if they feel this is not allowed or there is no opportunity. It is therefore helpful if:

- professionals are proactive
- the fact that a woman is having a termination of pregnancy is acknowledged and not avoided
- health professionals take responsibility for checking out how much a woman wants to know
- health professionals are fully informed about the system of care, including the procedure and the disposal of the remains of the pregnancy, so that questions can be confidently answered
- health professionals are briefed about the different ways a woman can interpret and react to early termination
- health professionals can develop good communication skills and build confidence in coping with women's emotional reactions.

❑ Organisational issues

There will be local variations in the service provided for the early termination of pregnancy within the NHS and also by private abortion clinics. The women in this study were all referred by their GP to the local hospital, where they were cared for in the day surgery unit or gynaecological ward.

Routine provision of counselling to be made available before and after termination

There is no opportunity provided locally in the NHS, for the women who need to, to discuss and explore the personal implications of the decision they are making with a professional who is independent of the decision-making process. It is likely that only a minority of women would take up this opportunity. At present women must take responsibility themselves for finding and funding counselling if they require it. Many women, arguably the most vulnerable, are unable to do this.

Similarly, post-termination counselling is unavailable for women for whom the termination itself may have presented difficulties or may have triggered other issues that become unmanageable. All women should have access to counselling help after the termination should they need it. Women need to know whom to contact and how.

Information about reactions post-termination

The information given to these women about likely postoperative reactions was limited and, from the women's point of view, poorly timed. They felt ill prepared. Women need accurate information in a form they can easily understand (verbal and written) about the likely physical and emotional consequences of termination. They need to know how their body is likely to react:

- how long the bleeding is likely to continue
- the indications of abnormal bleeding
- the likely onset of their next period and any changes they should expect
- contraceptive advice.

Disposal policy

In the hospital in this study the remains of the pregnancy following the termination are collected in a Sharps' box. It is accepted good practice that the remains of each pregnancy should be packaged individually (see SANDS 1995).

Increase in awareness between GPs and gynaecologists about the limitations of each other's role

It is common for the GP inaccurately to assume that the outpatient appointment routinely provides an opportunity for women to discuss their decision whilst the hospital doctors assume that women have discussed their decision with their GP. This misunderstanding is unhelpful to women. The provision of adequate counselling help available by choice but routinely offered would help overcome this problem.

GP follow-up care

GPs must be more proactive in providing appropriate follow-up care and recognise the potential physical and emotional consequences of termination of pregnancy. It is unhelpful for GPs to avoid the subject of the termination when women consult them.

■ Suggestions for further reading

Davies, V. (1991) *Abortion and Afterwards*, Bath, Ashgrove Press.
Neustatter, A. and Newson, G. (1986) *Mixed Feelings: The Experience of Abortion*, London, Pluto Press.

Chapter 4

Stillbirth, late miscarriage and termination of pregnancy

■ Introduction

❏ The local health care system

Antenatal care will normally have been shared between the GP, community midwife and hospital. The antenatal clinic, usually for those in the second and third trimesters, is in the main hospital. Ultrasound facilities are available in the clinic as well as the ultrasound department. If specialist prenatal ultrasound is indicated women will be referred to a regional centre. At the time of the study routine counselling help was unavailable to women making decisions about the termination of a pregnancy although the consultant could refer to the gynaecological social worker if he thought this appropriate.

Women whose baby is expected to be stillborn will be delivered on the maternity unit. The fetal death may be detected in hospital by a midwife or obstetrician or the woman may have approached her GP or community midwife with concerns about her pregnancy. Women whose pregnancies end during the second trimester because of miscarriage or termination will normally be cared for on the maternity unit but will be advised that they could also be cared for on the emergency ward. Normally, women who are having a second-trimester termination of pregnancy for reasons other than abnormality are referred to a private clinic.

Professionals differed in their views on when the maternity unit may be more appropriate for a woman than the emergency ward and on what the system is, but demonstrated a clear commitment to giving women a choice. It is thought that some women may prefer to be away from a maternity ward in close proximity to other mothers with healthy, crying babies. However, it is likely that women will not know what they are choosing between.

The hospital maternity unit includes the delivery suite and the antenatal and postnatal wards. A 'bereavement room' is available on the postnatal ward. It is pleasantly decorated and equipped with a double bed. This facility should be offered to all women on the maternity unit who deliver a baby who does not live. A hospital chaplain is always available, although

96

none of the women in this study wished to see one. At the time of this study the bereavement counsellor was extending her role to include the maternity unit but was not involved with any of the women in this study at the time of their loss.

In contrast to women whose baby is stillborn and are routinely visited by their GP and community midwife women who miscarry or whose pregnancy is terminated before 24 weeks have to indicate that they want the help of the primary health care team. Unlike hospital care the service that is provided after discharge from hospital is based on the gestation of the pregnancy rather than the needs of the woman.

❏ The women

Background information

Table 4.1 summarises the background information on the eight women in the study. The women varied in age from 25 to 34 years. All were in a stable relationship, considered their partner supportive and were leading settled lives. They varied in their reproductive history.

Table 4.1 Stillbirth, late miscarriage and termination: background information

	Age	Relationship	Occupation	Reproductive history
Mary	30	cohab/stable relationship	unemployed	first pregnancy
Sue	25	married	unemployed, previously shop assistant	TOP age 18
Jane	33	cohab/stable relationship	nurse manager	first pregnancy
Jenny	29	married	nurse	first pregnancy; history of infertility
Judith	30	married	nurse	third pregnancy; two early miscarriages
Linda	33	married	nurse	two TOPs aged 15 and 18; one child
Sheila	26	cohab/stable relationship	factory work	first pregnancy; reported difficulty in conceiving
Lisa	34	married	housewife, previously veterinary nurse	three children; treatment for endometriosis

TOP = termination of pregnancy.

Unusually, four of the women had a background in nursing and another was trained as a veterinary nurse. The women were recruited systematically and represent half the women who were admitted to hospital during the recruiting period of the project. There are two possible implications of the women having a nursing background. Firstly, they may be more committed to participate in research of this kind because they understand what it would involve and how it can help to improve services, but they may be more in sympathy with the values implicit in the system of care than the women who were not recruited. Secondly, staff may respond differently to a woman they consider to be 'one of them' and who speaks the same language. This can work to a woman's advantage in that she may have greater knowledge about the experience she is going through as well as knowing how to work the system to her advantage (like Linda) or to her disadvantage when it is assumed that she has knowledge and attributes she does not have (like Judith). There is no evidence that, in other respects, their nursing background meant the health care provided for them was significantly different.

Women's experience of the pregnancy

Apart from Lisa all the women were pleased to be pregnant. For Jenny it was a particularly special pregnancy, which she considered to be a miracle following infertility treatment. Table 4.2 summarises the women's experiences of the pregnancy.

Mary and Jane both had healthy pregnancies but became worried by lack of movement and, sensing something was wrong, contacted the maternity unit, where the fetal death was diagnosed. Sue was admitted for a planned, routine induction at 41 weeks, when no fetal heartbeat could be found. Although there was no clear explanation for the stillbirths apart from 'the cord was tightly round the neck', in none of these cases was professional intervention considered a factor in the cause of the stillbirth.

Jenny had bled early in the pregnancy. An abnormality (polyhydramnios) in her pregnancy was later diagnosed so the early signs of labour did not come as a surprise. At 23 weeks gestation twins were delivered; one lived for over an hour but the other was born dead and was registered as a stillbirth.

For Linda and Sheila severe fetal abnormalities were unexpectedly detected at routine scans at around 20 weeks gestation. Both abnormalities were incompatible with life, although this was only confirmed for Linda after the termination. Judith had not recognised the seriousness of the symptoms she experienced (watery discharge) until the registrar explained at the scan that there was no amniotic fluid. She reluctantly agreed to have a termination of pregnancy as she was advised. However, she had started to bleed before her admission to hospital for the termination. For these women it was likely that, had they continued with the pregnancy, they would not have reached term, so the termination merely hastened a process that would have occurred naturally at a later date.

Table 4.2 Stillbirth, late miscarriage and termination: women's experiences of the pregnancy

	Women's views about this pregnancy	Women's experiences of the pregnancy	Recognition of a problem with the pregnancy
Mary	planned and wanted	healthy, no problems	worried by lack of movement; consulted GP and went to maternity unit; fetal death diagnosed at scan
Sue	planned and wanted	healthy, no problems	admitted for routine induction; fetal death diagnosed at scan
Jane	planned and wanted	healthy, no problems	worried by lack of movement; went to maternity unit; fetal death diagnosed at scan
Jenny	planned and wanted; conception a miracle	difficult pregnancy because of pain, sickness and bleeding plus development of polyhydramnios	at diagnosis of polyhydramnios; one week later pains recognised as onset of labour
Judith	planned and wanted	anxiety because of previous miscarriage; bleeding in early pregnancy stopped; discharge leaking amniotic fluid but unrecognised	scan at 21 weeks revealed no amniotic fluid and confirmed nature of the discharge
Linda	planned and wanted	healthy, no problems	routine ultrasound revealed unexpected abnormality
Sheila	unplanned but wanted	healthy	routine ultrasound revealed unexpected abnormality
Lisa	unplanned and unexpected because of medical treatment; deeply distressed	only realised pregnant with weight gain	confirmation of pregnancy; fears that medication damaged baby unfounded; termination supported on grounds of mother's mental health

In contrast Lisa, an experienced mother of three, was being treated for endometriosis and thought she could not conceive. She only realised she might be pregnant when she started putting on weight and experiencing other symptoms. She was distraught. Although there were concerns that her medication may have damaged the fetus it was concluded that this was extremely unlikely and the termination was supported on the grounds of the risk to the mother's mental health. Because of her involvement with the hospital she was not referred to the private clinic, which would be normal practice for a pregnancy of this gestation (17 weeks).

Despite Lisa's reluctance to be pregnant and the relatively short time she had to get used to the idea, she, like the other women, had become very attached to her baby. Unlike the other women she had not, as they had done, begun to collect baby equipment, begun to think of names and involved family and friends in the pregnancy. Lisa had told no-one.

The categories of experience

Despite the obvious contrasts it seems appropriate to consider the second- and third-trimester losses together. Legal definitions apart there are clear differences in the experiences of miscarriage, stillbirth and termination. The women whose babies were stillborn or miscarried did not make the decision to end their baby's life, although they may have felt guilt and responsibility for their baby's death. Women deciding to terminate a pregnancy are faced with taking in complex information and making a decision they have to live with, often in a short period of time. In addition a baby born before 24 weeks gestation is unlikely to live whereas after the age of viability there is always the feeling that the baby had a chance.

But there are also similarities. All the women experienced labour (usually induced), delivery and its aftermath, as well as facing the ongoing physical, psychological and social adjustments to the end of their pregnancy and the loss of their baby. All the women were admitted to and, apart from one, cared for in the maternity unit. The health professionals they encountered were responsible for caring for them throughout this process.

Moreover it becomes clear that the boundaries between the different categories of experience are blurred and the terms, invested as they are with meaning, can be confusing or unhelpful. Table 4.3 contrasts the hospital's, the women's and the legal definitions. Two of the mid-trimester cases outlined above were similar but were defined differently. Jenny, diagnosed as suffering from polyhydramnios, went into spontaneous labour at 23 weeks: one twin was born dead; the other lived for over an hour. Her experience was defined as a miscarriage whilst she defined her loss as a stillbirth and was deeply offended when professionals referred to her 'miscarriage'. Judith, with oligohydramnios, took the advice she was given to terminate her pregnancy because of the abnormality. She was bleeding by the time she was admitted for the termination and her baby was macerated on delivery. She had strong feelings about termination and referred to her experience as a miscarriage whilst the professionals referred to it as a termination.

Table 4.3   Stillbirth, late miscarriage and termination: different definitions

	Hospital definition of experience as presented to researchers	Woman's definition	Gestation (weeks)	Place cared for	Legal definition
Mary	stillbirth	stillbirth	36	maternity unit	stillbirth
Sue	stillbirth	stillbirth	41	maternity unit	stillbirth
Jane	stillbirth	stillbirth	39	maternity unit	stillbirth
Jenny	miscarriage	stillbirth	23	maternity unit	miscarriage and neonatal death
Judith	TFA	TFA	23	maternity unit	TFA
Linda	TFA	miscarriage	21	maternity unit	TFA/miscarriage
Sheila	TFA	TFA	19/21	maternity unit	TFA
Lisa	TFA	TFA	17	emergency ward	termination on grounds of mother's mental health

TFA = termination for abnormality.

With the exception of the consultant, a thread of confusion about the reason for the termination of Lisa's pregnancy ran through the discussions with all the participants of her case. Lisa, and the staff caring for her, defined her experience as a termination for abnormality whereas the termination was agreed to on the grounds of the mother's mental health. As this confusion clearly illustrates, some women and health professionals re-define the category of a woman's experience in a way that makes sense to and suits them.

In addition it cannot be assumed that experiences which are defined as the same are similar. A termination of pregnancy when the baby has an abnormality incompatible with life and the pregnancy may well have not reached full term is different for both parents and staff from a termination for what many might consider a minor disability.

In practice many health professionals, particularly on the maternity unit, do not appear to make distinctions between the different categories of experience. For example, in informal discussions with midwives, all the involuntary losses occurring on the maternity unit were referred to as stillbirths and distinctions are not made in the quality of the care that is offered. The basis of their relationship with the woman is that they are losing a baby and not the gestation of the baby or whether the pregnancy was terminated or the reason for it. Perhaps the less categorical and stigmatising terms of intrauterine death and induction are more helpful terms to use.

❑ Professionals' views of stillbirth, late miscarriage and termination

All the health professionals interviewed recognised the significance of still-birth and second-trimester miscarriage and termination. The desire to help, to make it better and to take away the pain was implicit in many health professionals' views of the nature of later pregnancy loss. There was a generosity of spirit and a recognition of the human tragedy involved.

The later gestation of the pregnancy was seen by many health professionals as making it worse because the woman would have formed a stronger attachment to the baby, who would be bigger and more fully developed, she would have gone through labour for nothing and the pregnancy would be more public. Conversely, others thought these factors, in contrast to early miscarriage, made later loss more immediate, obvious and accessible and therefore more able to be shared. A GP, in talking about one of his patients, summed up several professionals' views on the difference in attachment:

> I think these are the most emotionally charged situations. Early loss in pregnancy is terrible but I think once it's 22 weeks it's just getting worse and I think maximum understanding and time is what she needs.

Whilst acknowledging that they thought later loss was worse the professionals were anxious to stress that they did not dismiss the potential impact of early loss and described it as a difference in intensity of reaction.

A consultant stressing that 'the physical reality makes it worse' thought that later loss was more difficult for women and therefore more distressing for health professionals. Behind this comment is the central issue that later pregnancy loss cannot be avoided for what it is. Unlike with early miscarriage and termination it is impossible for either women or health professionals to present the experience as an illness with little or nothing to do with pregnancy. The women will labour and deliver their baby and must be cared for accordingly.

It was generally recognised that the experience of termination for abnormality had added dimensions of difficulty for women because they were faced with making a difficult decision and the responsibility for ending the pregnancy, as one midwife commented:

> Usually it's a wanted baby and it's a baby that is alive and well, albeit with some abnormality and the parents are having to make the decision to actually end the pregnancy. So basically they are terminating the baby's life, as it were... with a stillbirth, yes it is a

wanted baby and it's died but it's beyond your control. It's not actually something you actually went out and said 'Right. That's it.' ...I think they have probably got more guilt on it... no matter how they rationalise it.

As their experience of their health care illustrates (see below) there is little evidence that women who had a termination of pregnancy were judged adversely, contrary to the women's expectations. A few professionals commented that they did not approve of termination of pregnancy in the second trimester other than for reasons of abnormality. It is unlikely that the professionals in this study would be involved in caring for women whose pregnancy was terminated for other reasons in the second trimester. Locally, NHS care for these women would be provided at a private abortion clinic.

Many professionals commented on the relative frequency and therefore normality of early loss compared with the infrequency of later loss, as this registrar commented:

I think the differentiation between a mid-trimester or an early pregnancy loss and a late pregnancy loss is – people seeing... You know, we see hundreds of miscarriages and we are very dismissive of them and I think that is wrong. I don't know that there should be a distinction between the two.

One experienced GP pointed out that, in 25 years of practice, he had never before had a patient who had miscarried at 23 weeks gestation. For one midwife there was a gap of seven years between her involvement in the diagnosis of a fetal death in utero. It is common for health professionals to lack exposure to stillbirth, late miscarriage or termination and therefore to feel inadequate and lacking in confidence in their understanding of the complexity of the experience and in their professional skills.

❏ Overall evaluation of care

Table 4.4 summarises the women's perceptions of hospital care and Table 4.7 summarises the women's perceptions of care after discharge from hospital. The women on the whole felt extremely well cared for in hospital and thought highly of the staff, whom they said had gone out of their way to help them. Two women were less satisfied with their care. It was difficult for staff responsible for their health care to establish an effective relationship with them. Mary was critical of the help that she was offered and kept all professionals at a distance. Lisa was not critical but actively rejected help of any kind. It is hard not to draw the conclusion that she was punishing herself for a decision she quickly came to regret. Both Lisa and Mary were difficult women to help. Neither established a close relationship with staff

Table 4.4   Stillbirth, late miscarriage and termination: women's perceptions of hospital care

| | Diagnosis/decision-making | Preparation before induction/delivery | Management of labour | Management of delivery | Handling/management of baby | Management of consent for post-mortem | Management post-delivery | | Management of discharge | Management of arrange for disposal |
							Delivery suite	Post-natal ward bereavement room		
Mary	2	2	4	2	4	4	4	–	1	2
Sue	1	4	2	2	1	3	1	–	4	1
Jane	5	4	1	1	1	4	1	1	1	1
Jenny	1	1	1	1	1	–	1	–	1	1
Judith	4	1	1	1	1	3	1	–	1	1
Linda	2	4	1	2	1	4	1	5	5	1
Sheila	1	1	1	1	2	–	1	1	1	1
Lisa	5	5	5	5	4	5	3*	–	3	5

* NB: cared for on the emergency ward and not in the maternity unit.

1 = very helpful
2 = helpful
3 = neither helpful nor unhelpful
4 = unhelpful
5 = very unhelpful

during their hospital admission. On reflection we can speculate that if Mary had been helped to prepare herself more effectively for the delivery of her stillborn baby and Lisa had been helped to make a more considered decision about her pregnancy things would have been different, but it is easy to be wise after the event.

The women's views of care after discharge from hospital are less positive reflecting the more haphazard quality and availability of care in the community as well as the difficulty primary health care staff face in picking up the pieces after such an intense experience in hospital. The operation of a more rigid divide at 24 weeks gestation meant that services such as the community midwife were only available to the women whose babies were stillborn.

These issues will be discussed in detail as the different aspects of care are considered in turn.

■ Hospital care: diagnosis and decision-making

❏ Stillbirth and late miscarriage

Sue's experience

> she took the blood pressure and... then she went to do a heart monitor. And she couldn't find a heart beat. But she said it could have been the fact that the baby was in an awkward position. She said it could have been the machine so we went up another ward and tried another one up there... The doctor that did the scan sort of went away and said he wanted a second opinion. At that stage I thought something is wrong... I always thought that the baby was in an awkward position. I though they might have to do an emergency caesarean or something. And then another midwife come back, and she did a heart monitor and couldn't get nothing then and she went away and the consultant came with his under consultant and the midwife and a student nurse that was training. And they sort of did another scan and then he turned round and said 'I'm very sorry.' And that's when I knew something was wrong.

> He just said there was no heartbeat. He said, 'I can't feel a heart beat, there's no life. I'm not seeing anything going on.' And that was just it. And I mean I broke down and Peter broke down... I mean at first I was dead set against having an induction... I wanted a caesarean to get it out of the way. I didn't want nothing to do with it.

> He turned round and said, 'We're going to have to induce labour. You can have all the painkillers you're going to need. Which means once this baby is delivered you can go home quite quick. If you have a caesarean he said you'll be in hospital a bit longer.'

I mean I was in shock and everything and I wanted just to get rid of it, I wanted nothing to do with it.

Diagnosis

The diagnosis that something is wrong is usually unpredictable and unplanned. It is always a sensitive and emotionally charged event for all involved, with great potential for misunderstanding, adding to the distress. It may be difficult for staff to give the information if they have strong feelings about wanting to 'make it all right/better' and it is often hard for women and their partners to take in the information they are given.

Despite the inevitable involvement of additional, often unknown, staff and transfer to a different room or ultrasound machine Mary, Sue and Jenny, whose babies were stillborn or miscarried and who were cared for by senior midwives or doctors (registrar or consultant), valued the clear and sensitive explanations they had been given and appreciated the compassion of the staff involved. They were reassured that they would be given as much pain relief as they needed and options in their care were discussed with them, including the opportunity to go home before induction and seeing their baby. Whilst decisions were not necessarily made, the opportunities for choice were raised and time created to think about what they might want.

Jane's experience

In contrast Jane was shocked by the reaction of the midwife who she felt was unable to contain her own distress at the diagnosis and was therefore unable to offer her and her husband effective help. In Jane's words:

this midwife was unable to cope. She... you could see... when I was waiting to see a doctor when I was down in Outpatient waiting to be scanned. I could hear her say, 'I knew! I knew! I knew!' You know she was hysterical. I could hear her... She'd been in the delivery suite and she'd come down with us. And we were in a doctor's office and I could hear her saying it. And then we went up to the ward and I was then her patient I guess and she was dealing with me and she had a checklist which she worked through... she was the person who told us we could take her home but she said about maceration and everything and... What she was trying to do... was I wanted to have a caesarean section at that stage and she wanted to make me feel better.

Jane was led to believe her labour would be quick and her baby macerated, neither of which proved to be the case. The midwife recognised her own discomfort and inexperience in this situation and had been troubled by it. She worried that she prolonged Jane's agony by delaying confirmation of the diagnosis. This diagnosis was complicated by scan machines that did not work, transfer from the maternity ward to the antenatal clinic and the involvement of different doctors. Nevertheless the options in her care were discussed, albeit in rather an abrupt manner, and Jane was grateful for her encouragement to go home before admission to hospital and her preparation in thinking about seeing the baby. Six months later Jane recognised that whilst the midwife found the diagnosis difficult and in her view should not take on this task she had offered constructive help but, as the weak link in their care, had become the focus of their anger at the loss of their baby.

❑ Termination for abnormality

Making the decision: Linda's experience

> I was plodding along as usual with my pregnancy when I went for my scan at 21 weeks.

An abnormality was detected at a routine scan when Linda was 21 weeks pregnant. She was referred to a specialist unit where a severe abnormality was diagnosed. Over the following week she discussed her baby's prognosis with her obstetric consultant, with a senior paediatric registrar and with the specialist over the phone. Linda and her husband were very distressed. In a short period of time they had to absorb a lot of new information and work out what more they needed to find out. They each latched on to and interpreted differently the information they had been given and needed time together to talk. They returned for a second appointment at the specialist unit:

> they were very helpful and everybody said that they would support any decision we made. But obviously it was for us to make that decision, which was very difficult. I think we had half made it anyway but just the final sort of information confirmed that was what we felt the best thing was for the baby... I think we'd spent the week talking about it on and off and we'd sort of weighed up the fact of what life would be like for the baby which was our main concern.

> What would we be putting the baby through? Would we have been putting it through that because we didn't want to make the decision at this stage? Or were we doing it because we felt the baby would have a good quality of life? And we didn't. We didn't feel that he would have done at all. You know we were told that he may have needed an operation fairly soon after birth. I think if that had been the case and that would have been it then I think we probably would have gone ahead because at that stage, though they know about it at the time, they don't remember it. And we felt we could cope with that together. But with the outlook being that he would have had an awful lot more

operations, numerous stays in hospital and the specialist said that these babies don't... often grow up into adults... that confirmed that we felt what we were doing was right for him. And also for our son because we had to think of him as well, what he would have gone through.

we talked about it a lot on the train coming home... and felt that that was the decision we had to make and really we wanted to sort of get it – sounds awful – get it over with. You know, go through the process as soon as possible because time wasn't on my side.

The ultrasound scan

The abnormality was unexpectedly detected at routine ultrasound scan for all three women, although Judith had experienced worrying symptoms which she had ignored. Inevitably, all the women were shocked that something was wrong and took time to take in the information, half believing it would be all right before coming to realise it would not. Judith describes how she realised it had all gone wrong:

In the scan she said she could see a fetal heart. And then she said that there is no fluid around the baby. And that really didn't mean anything to me at the time... she said 'It's a good job that you have come today – to get this all sorted out.' And so she videoed a few pictures, that sort of thing... I said, 'Well I'd been losing this discharge stuff, do you think it's that? And I soaked a whole sanitary towel with it last night.' And she said, 'That's not right at all.' She said, 'I'll phone up the antenatal clinic to see if they want to see you.' So we waited and they wanted to see us at the end of their antenatal clinic. And I thought at the time you know, at 21 weeks you know there's a baby there. Something can be done to preserve it. When I got home suddenly it hit me, the realisation that my waters had broke, the waters had gone and there was no hope for the pregnancy.

When Judith saw the registrar he explained why there might be a lack of amniotic fluid and that she probably needed a termination. He arranged an appointment with the consultant in a few days time after the Bank Holiday weekend for another scan, which was for her benefit. He thought she needed time for the news to sink in. She was left worrying about the implications of having a termination.

The women reported that the sonographers explained the need for referral to a doctor in general terms and, where asked directly, gave honest answers. Judith and Sheila were seen promptly by a senior doctor (consultant or registrar) and given clear explanations. To Linda's regret a doctor was unavailable at the time of the scan to discuss the result with her in person, although telephone contact was offered. It was left to the sonographer to tell her she had an appointment at a London hospital the following day. She worked out for herself that something must be very wrong and realised how serious when she arrived at the hospital to discover the appointment was in a specialist unit and not the ultrasound department.

Discussion with the consultant

> This Dr Jones he don't muck about. He told me straight I was going to lose him... I'd sooner know straight than be mucked about. 'Cos I know some doctors they go round the bush and still it leads to the same thing in the end doesn't it? Sheila

All the women had at least one appointment with a consultant to discuss the diagnosis and the decision that had to be made. Explanations and scans were willingly repeated and appointments arranged so that partners could be present. Considerable effort was made to contact one woman's partner at work. On the whole the women valued the level of concern that was expressed, the straightforward way in which difficult information was conveyed and the opportunities provided to ask questions and have them answered. They were also given time to take in the information and were not rushed into making decisions or an early admission to hospital. Their wishes were respected.

A consultant describes the purpose of his appointment with Linda:

> my job is really to help her with the decision she has to take once the abnormality is discovered. And basically I would outline the possibilities of what was likely to show up at the next scan and then talk to her about what we can offer her, what's available so that she has a clear insight into what is available, being quite realistic. This is on the practical side of everything... available for the baby, what can be done at delivery, what it actually means going through and what then if she opts for a termination, what that involves, what that means, how long she'll have to wait, what procedure is undertaken and what she is going to feel like afterwards and the risks of depression and all that. I go through all those things with her so at least when she goes for the final scan she has already got in her mind some idea of what to expect and what is going to happen. And I... don't take any role in the decision making unless she asks me to. I give her the facts.

However, helping people make complex decisions is not purely a matter of giving them information but also of enabling them to make choices that are right for them. Often it is only possible to offer a limited degree of choice. Judith remained confused about the extent of choice she had:

He was very good in a sense in that he just took the decision right out of my hands... He said, 'There is absolutely no future with this pregnancy... it's not a question of will you have a termination it's when you can come in to be induced.' So he said it like that. And then they turned the tables really and said that the decision's up to you and if you want to carry on with the pregnancy you can... I think he was strongly saying that no way can you go on with it but... it's your decision... he was very sympathetic. He told us exactly what was going on and he said if he was in my shoes he wouldn't hesitate for a termination.

Judith remained troubled by the decision she made to end her pregnancy. By the time she was admitted to hospital she was bleeding and her baby was macerated on delivery. She referred to her experience as a miscarriage, which by then it was.

Despite finding her appointment with the consultant helpful in all other respects Linda was upset by what she considered inappropriate comments:

He agreed we had a very difficult decision to make and only we could make it. He weighed up the pros and cons, explained the procedure if we went ahead, explained about pain relief... and in that sense it was helpful... and if we decided, it could be done at our convenience, when we were ready.

I've asked not to see the consultant again because he made a couple of remarks to me which I felt were very unnecessary. He seemed very nice. I mean I hadn't met him before but he did say to me did I realise that I would be saving the NHS an awful lot of money. I thought that was very unnecessary... I was sort of in between making the decision. Luckily my husband wasn't there... he probably would have hit him... And he also, which I didn't tell my husband, he also told me to ignore my husband, it's my decision. I did say, 'Oh no, it's our decision.' But I felt those were very unnecessary remarks and very uncaring, very thoughtless.

He'd had the letter from the specialist unit to say what the problem was and everything. And I think it was just... I mean it was nice to be able to go and see him. It was a voluntary thing. I didn't have to go but I thought well that's nice, you feel that there is support there, people are understanding what you are going through, it is a very difficult time. And I thought well you know any sort of information or support we can get is all to the good. But when I came away I didn't feel I got that at all.

The need for more information and discussion

Linda and Judith used the interval between the diagnosis and making the decision to seek further information either from books or from an expert known personally to them. They were resourceful women and could access the expertise they needed but even so Judith was clearly unprepared for the reality of the termination and was admitted to hospital not fully appreciating that she had to go through labour. Sheila, who was less well educated, trusted implicitly the advice she was given and did not need to seek further information.

None of these women had access to other sources of professional help during this time. The primary health care teams were not involved and knew of the diagnosis only after the termination had taken place. However good the explanation about the diagnosis, the process and the likely implications for the woman, a consultant appointment does not offer the opportunity for a thorough exploration of the woman's feelings about the termination and preparation for it. Routine referral to a specialist counsellor would provide this opportunity. Judith, for example, had strong views about termination and remained troubled by her decision to terminate her pregnancy. These women managed by making good use of the resources available to them. Other more vulnerable women may be unable to do so.

❑ Termination: the lack of opportunity for a more measured decision

Lisa had ignored the early signs of pregnancy because her periods had always been erratic and she was taking medication for a gynaecological condition. She was about 14 weeks pregnant when her GP confirmed her pregnancy. She never received notification of the appointment which was made for her with the consultant obstetrician, who knew her well. She had not planned to be pregnant and was worried about the effect the drugs she had taken would have on her baby. Another outpatient appointment was made for her but with a different consultant because time was running out.

Lisa found the consultant sympathetic and thoughtful. She had a scan and saw the screen, which she found distressing. Afterwards she had the opportunity for discussion with the consultant but was too upset to think of any questions. The consultant realised she had not told her husband and suggested she did so. She agreed with the consultant to make up her mind by the following day and was given the number of the labour ward to ring if she decided to go ahead with the termination.

The consultant, who was under the impression that Lisa had already decided to go ahead with the termination but thought she might change her mind, was clear that the risk of abnormality was minimal but that a termination could be supported on the grounds that the pregnancy was unexpected and that Lisa was anxious and depressed. He thought this had been made clear to Lisa. Lisa briefly discussed this appointment with the GP, told her husband and made the arrangements with the hospital to be admitted in two days time. She describes her feelings about making the decision:

> I always had such strong feelings about never ever having an abortion. It comes hard then when you've got to make a decision, should I? Shouldn't I? And I know for a fact that if I hadn't had the other children that I would have gone ahead with it whatever. I also thought about the baby afterwards. What would be wrong with it? Is it going to have a miserable existence? I remember in the end my head was just about ready to explode I think... trying to take everything in... When I did find out that I was pregnant was just... I was waking up every night and I was having nightmares that I'd stabbed a baby and to me that is what I'd done. All I was doing was murdering a baby. Now I have nightmares that when I wake up I can hear a baby crying and I can't find the baby.

> The gynaecologist... asked me what my husband thought... and said you really need to talk to somebody else... about it. And even then I didn't want to. I didn't want anyone else to know I was even thinking about doing what I did... He [her husband] was quite supportive. But at the end of the day it came back to the same thing that everybody else had said to me. It's got to be your decision. So it's got to be that choice whether or not to let it live. That's the worst feeling in the world. And it's me... and although they actually caused it to go away it's my fault because it was me that said yes.

> I so much wanted someone to say, 'Have it.' I told my mum... She was the only person really that said, 'If you want it, have it. We'll help you.'... But then at the end of the day they're getting older... I really wanted someone to either say, 'yes you should have it' or 'no you really shouldn't have it'. But nobody said that. Everybody said it's got to be your decision.

> [On the day of her admission to hospital] I sat at the golf course for an hour and a half because I couldn't go, I couldn't... I didn't want anyone to come with me, I didn't want anybody there, I didn't want anybody to see what I was doing. And... I nearly drove home so many times during that hour and a half.

Lisa regretted the decision she had made.

Confusion characterised the confirmation of Lisa's pregnancy and the consultant appointment. The consultant was helpfully slotting in an extra patient because the appointment was for a request for termination. Lisa appeared to the consultant to be very clear about what she wanted whereas she was undecided, acutely distressed and felt rushed into making a decision she later regretted. There was no opportunity for counselling. Although Lisa was reluctant to discuss her decision with anyone because she felt so ashamed and may not have accepted help from an outsider, especially if she would have had to initiate the contact, a skilled specialist counsellor may have been able to help her explore the very strong feelings she had about what she was doing and to make a more measured decision.

■ Hospital care: labour and delivery

❑ Introduction: the maternity unit

In general the women received high-quality care on the maternity unit (Table 4.5). They were cared for either by very experienced senior midwives or more junior midwives who had expressed an interest in this area of work. They would not describe themselves as specialists but clearly had or were developing particular areas of expertise. Whilst often finding it a stressful, demanding and sometimes frightening part of their work they clearly communicated to the women a degree of comfort with the experience and viewed assisting a woman to deliver a dead or dying baby as an important and positive part of their job.

It must not be assumed that all midwives on the unit have developed the same degree of expertise or comfort with the experience. For example, one woman described an encounter with a midwife who had the specific task to help her wash and move to a different room: 'She could not look me in the eye or look at my baby.'

All the women were cared for at a time when the unit was described by the midwives as 'quiet' or 'not that busy'. The midwives were able to give the women their full attention and were not responsible for delivering another woman at the same time, a situation that was described by several midwives as 'horrendous' in demanding an almost impossible switch of emotions. In addition, because of the length and timing of their labour and delivery, several women were cared for by the same midwife for more than one shift. There was the opportunity for a close and trusting relationship to develop. These circumstances cannot always prevail, as the midwife who cared for Linda suggested:

> I think she was cared for well but I think luck played a huge part in it. I think if you are lucky you come on the ward when... somebody can spend all that time with you... I was talking to her. If she needed me I was there. We made facilities available for her husband and all those sorts of things. But that's the best we'd ever get and it's not often achieved. So for Linda I felt very happy... But had it been another night, with a lot of activity in the labour ward, it could have been very different. It often is unfortunately.

Table 4.5 Stillbirth, late miscarriage and termination: labour and delivery

	Labour induced	Approx. time from onset of induction/ rupture of membranes to delivery (hours)	Pain relief		ERPC	Women's views		Professional views
			Diamorphine	Epidural		Expectation that labour would be quicker and less painful	Views of delivery	
Mary	✓	9	✓	✓	I week later	✓	pain relief always too little and too late; felt completely abandoned	woman low pain threshold and frightened of the pain; midwife constantly popping in and out
Sue	✓	32	✓	✓	–	✓	'high as a kite'; didn't know what was happening to her	woman very detached and difficult to relate to; a difficult delivery; registrar feared decapitating baby
Jane	✓	33	✓	✓	–	✓	felt privileged to have given birth; enjoyed the delivery because she could do it.	midwife delighted at normal delivery
Jenny	–	4	pethidine, gas and oxygen		–	✓	felt calm, 'an amazing experience for both of us'	the woman was able to labour and deliver in the way she wanted
Judith	✓	24	✓	–	✓	✓	labour longer than anticipated but delivery not difficult	an easy person to care for because of emotional openness and knowledge about labour and delivery
Linda	✓	30	✓	For ERPC	✓	✓	delivery 'brutish tug-o'-war'; a dreadful smell	midwife had called registrar who then delivered the baby, which she regretted
Sheila	✓	40	✓	✓	–	no	relatively easy	long and difficult labour
Lisa	✓	12	✓	–	✓	✓	felt alone and abandoned on her own	woman was very distressed, midwife couldn't do anything to help

There are good working relationships between midwives and doctors based on respect for each other's separate areas of expertise. Most of the senior obstetricians have recently trained in breaking bad news, which they said they found extremely helpful. A striking feature of the maternity unit is the midwifery manager and the high esteem in which she is held by the midwives and doctors alike. She was consistently described as approachable, sensitive, caring to her staff and committed to providing an excellent service for women. She has taken a particular interest in the care provided for women whose babies die and has improved the guidelines and support available for the midwives. She makes herself personally available to her staff when needed. In addition the general manager for the unit is perceived as approachable, flexible and supportive to the midwives. His personal concern for the staff when particularly distressing events occurred was frequently commented on. The culture of the maternity unit is therefore supportive.

❏ The place for labour and delivery

The maternity unit

All these women were admitted to the maternity unit and all apart from Lisa were cared for there. Staff are often concerned about where is the best place for a woman delivering a dead or dying baby to be cared for and worry that she may feel shunted out of the way in a side room or about the proximity of healthy crying babies and happy mothers. The concerns are often a reflection of discomfort about the proximity of birth and death as well as uncertainty about the meaning of the event for some women, uncertainty about the importance of gestation and the significance that should be attached to termination and the reason for it. Consideration of where a woman should be cared for begs the question of how her experience is defined and clarifies the lack of clear boundaries between the different experiences.

Several of the midwives expressed concern at what they considered to be poor facilities; the room was particularly hot or lacked the private facilities they thought appropriate in such circumstances. Whilst the proximity to healthy babies was an issue for some of the women postnatally and the personal distaste for the decorations in the room became the focus for one woman's anger at her long and difficult labour, the place where these women laboured and delivered their babies was not an issue for them. The relationship they had with their midwife and the fact that they felt psychologically well cared for and 'wanted' appeared to dissipate any concerns they may have had about being in the wrong place or out of order, as Linda described: 'They gave us a room, the last room, but didn't make us feel they were putting us out of the way but that it was for our own benefit and privacy.'

The delivery of the baby on the maternity unit can be interpreted positively by women as confirmation of their role as mother or negatively in terms of the loss of their baby. It was especially helpful for Jenny whose twin daughters were delivered at 23 weeks gestation. It confirmed and legitimated the existence of her babies, as she described:

> I was so pleased that we had been on the delivery suite because that's where you go to have your baby. It meant an awful lot being in there. I thought... in fact [the midwife] said when we went back on the Wednesday, 'Will it upset you coming here with your babies?' Well it didn't and it wasn't upsetting really hearing other babies cry because that's where our babies were born, they were born there.

The emergency ward

Lisa's pregnancy was terminated at 17 weeks gestation. On admission to the maternity unit she was given the choice of staying there or being cared for on the emergency ward. She was in a distressed state, unable to make up her mind and did not know what she was choosing:

> It just seemed all decisions. If there had been somewhere, a particular somewhere that you go, that you didn't have to be asked... It seems such a small decision but on top of everything else it isn't. Do I want to be up here? Do I want to hear babies crying? Do I want to be downstairs? It meant nothing to me... I knew the maternity unit but I had no idea what ward G was about... I didn't know it was an emergency ward. I didn't have a clue... Obviously the nurses have dealt with things like that before but... it's not what they do if you see what I mean.

On reflection Lisa regretted choosing to be cared for on the emergency ward and wished she had not been given the choice.

Labour and delivery do not normally take place on the emergency ward. Lisa describes her views of what it was like for the staff:

> It must be hard for them I think especially for the nurses. I felt really sorry for them because they're dealing with umpteen other things. They are dealing with Mrs So and So along the corridor and Mrs So and So up the other way and then they remember 'I'd just better pop in and try and see how she is.' And you can see that they are like torn. They are trying to do 50,000 other things at once... They were lovely... I couldn't fault them in any way. But they didn't know how to deal with it.

The nurse caring for her thought the emergency ward was not the best place for her to be cared for. The consultant thought the maternity unit offered the most appropriate care but that it was important to give women the choice not to be near crying babies. Both emphasised that the emergency ward was very busy. Another consultant expressed his concern that women were cared for on the emergency ward:

> you don't go to the plumber if your car is broken. If you've got a baby being delivered who do you get to do it? A midwife. They are looking after people in pain and delivering all the time – whether the baby happens to be this big or this big I don't think it really matters particularly.

The consequences of the choice that Lisa made appear to be quite profound. There was confusion about who had responsibility for administering the pessaries that would bring about the termination. This was discussed in front of Lisa and in the event a series of different staff came down from the maternity unit to do this. The nurse caring for her disappeared out of the room in response to another patient's demands at the point of delivery. She delivered alone and when the nurse appeared was told not to look at the baby. She feared the baby had been born alive. She did see the baby and her views on disposal were sought but the arrangements were muddled, resulting in Lisa making a complaint to the hospital. There is no doubt that Lisa was very upset, as her nurse describes:

> I think she was so shocked by everything and I think there were rather difficult social circumstances as well... She came in completely on her own. She didn't have anybody with her, she didn't have her mum with her or her husband with her or anybody else with her. And really most of the time she was on the verge of tears. She avoided eye contact and didn't speak very much and, you know, it made me feel quite awkward because I didn't really know – I could see she was really upset but I didn't know what to say to make it any better because there wasn't anything I could say. So that all I could say to her was, 'I know you are really upset and there is nothing that I can say that will make you feel any better.'

Had she been cared for on the maternity unit by staff with more experience of these issues it is less likely that these problems would have arisen.

❏ Preparation for labour

All the women valued the opportunities they were given to discuss the management of their labour and delivery throughout the duration of their health care. There was an ongoing process of discussion, which started with the consultant or registrar and midwife at the diagnosis and continued on admission to hospital and throughout labour.

However, it is difficult to prepare women adequately for the experience and their expectations did not match the reality. Five of the six women whose labour was induced, including the one woman who had previously given birth to a baby at term, were shocked at the length and pain of their labour. Sheila appeared very accepting of what her consultant described as a long, emotionally demanding and exhausting labour. One of the women delivered her baby nine hours after the onset of the induction but four took 30 hours or more (see Table 4.5 above). They all said they had been led to believe labour would be quick because their pregnancy was not full term or because their baby had died.

The value of accurate and honest information in helping women to cope with the experience is illustrated by Jane's experience. She had understood that her labour would be less difficult and shorter than normal because her baby had died. She found her labour extremely difficult to cope with initially but then began to talk to her midwife:

> How quick will it be? She said, 'Well you've got to expect it to be a long time.' And she said, 'You won't be having your baby before this time tomorrow at the earliest.' Which was like 24 hours, which was much more realistic. And then we started dealing with it and in fact that 36 hours that I was in there for before she was born was incredibly valuable time. Preparation, getting used to it; it was talking to people, crying with people, being with people. And I feel very very privileged to have given birth too... which is funny... stillbirth isn't a wholly negative experience.

She also said she had been told her baby would be macerated which was not the case:

> I've forgotten her exact words but she said that she would be very macerated... every other midwife after that... said, 'No, she's not been dead for very long. She's going to be perfect.' But that was my major fear throughout labour. I was frightened about seeing her, what she was going to look like.

❑ Experiences of labour and delivery

Linda, an easy person to care for: termination for abnormality

The midwife described Linda as an easy person to care for because she was an emotionally open, receptive, knowledgeable and competent person. The midwife described how she cared for her:

> One of the things I think she was worried about was whether the baby would breathe when it was born because obviously it could have done.

And I think because of the amount of drugs we used that wasn't a problem... I let Linda potter about and let her get herself prepared mentally. She wanted to have a freshen up and all that sort of thing. And then when she was ready she rang the bell and I went down and started all the procedure for her. It was quite a long night really. We increased the drugs quite a lot. It's a big dose and it took a long time to do the work really. So we progressed through the night slowly. Often it's that way, you know, the cervix just won't open and then suddenly it all happened... I elected to stay on and support her through that. She had pain relief started at midnight and that worked very very well and that is all part of the relaxation, everything helps.

Linda described what happened from her point of view:

I started with the pessaries at nine and then the one I had just after that, the baby stopped moving, which in hindsight I'm glad about because I feel that he didn't have to go through labour and the delivery process. That he was in there, he was peaceful, he was warm and comfortable, you know, was there... It just sort of went on and on really, which is nobody's fault. I mean it's just the way it is really. They say they'd give you five pessaries, three hours apart. And then they say that they usually like to rest you overnight, which I didn't want... once it started I wanted to carry on... I was getting tightenings, there wasn't anything particularly significant happening at all. So they then put up a drip. That was about ten, half ten at night. And then the pains, you know, they did start then and then they put a diamorphine drip infusion up as well which eventually when it worked was very nice. It took away the physical pain and then I suppose about sevenish the midwife that was looking after me then had a look to see how far I had dilated and sort of said that I was ready to push.

Jane, a proud delivery: stillbirth

Jane was eventually able to use the time she was in labour positively to prepare for the birth of her baby. She describes what happened:

And once I actually got into it I really enjoyed it because I could do it. And Pauline [friend] was sort of... and the midwife were just... I had my feet up on their hips and they were just keeping me going and Graham [partner] was with me and that was brilliant. I was being fed lots of rich honey between each contraction and she was born at 1:37. She was perfect. There was nothing wrong with her... We will probably never know what was wrong with her. I felt so proud.

Jane attributed her ability to deliver her baby in this way to the support and encouragement the midwife gave her. It was a positive experience for the midwife too:

> And I think on this occasion it was really good, you know I tried very hard to be quiet and just listened to what they had to say. Just get the general feel of their views and that is difficult at times. You know, you have to be very open with them and if you are feeling unsure you actually have to share it with them. 'I'm not sure really is this what you want.'

> But the actual delivery all I can say is that Jane and her partner were just so thrilled to see the baby's head – and they were delighted because she had a normal delivery. Previously we had discussed that at great length, you know, that was really one of her big worries during the delivery: how was she going to cope, which is normal again.

> She wasn't sure, she didn't want to hold it immediately. I think she just wanted it left, just to see her reactions really, to see how she felt at the time… When the baby was delivered the baby was beautiful. I actually was so – when the baby was born – was so delighted that she had pushed this baby out. And she was and her partner was. I remember that was a tremendous hurdle. I found myself so delighted that I actually congratulated her for pushing this baby out… I tried to treat it as if it was all a normal birth. A normal birth and a live baby, just that the baby was asleep.

Sue, a difficult labour and traumatic delivery: stillbirth

Sue had a long and difficult labour and a traumatic delivery. She found the pain hard to tolerate and was given high levels of pain relief. Her reactions at the time appeared to the staff caring for her as unnaturally humorous and they worried about her future welfare. The registrar delivered her baby with forceps and feared the baby would be decapitated in the process.

The registrar saw her when she requested a caesarean section:

> She was very upset… upset and detached really and I don't think at the time she fully grasped what was happening to her… She was fed up with the pain and was testing the generosity of everybody. We had a chat at that time about the best possible option really in trying to convince her that we should push on towards a vaginal delivery… I don't think you could say it was a genuine choice because I think everybody was quite strongly persuading her to continue having the induction, vaginally. So I couldn't say it was an unbiased discussion at that time… I am worried that perhaps she will always feel very bitter about that, that we twisted her arm and forced her to have a normal

delivery, which was traumatic for her. It was unfortunate and completely unforeseen and unpredictable.

The midwife's view

> She very early adopted the role of being here in illness and drugged... it was as if... she was ill in hospital, not that she was going to give birth to her baby... It was terribly difficult because... she cried quite a lot, which was obviously traumatic. And we talked about how... this was her first baby. The fact the baby was dead didn't take away from the fact that this was their first child and she had sad feelings and so on and so forth... I asked her to name the baby and they wouldn't name the baby the name they had chosen for it. They wanted to save that name for one that was alive. And I tried to pinpoint her through the day about thinking for a name for the baby, I wanted to try to focus them on the baby.

Sue described the support from the midwife:

> She was ever so nice. She was the one that told Peter when she came in on Tuesday when she started us off... she said, 'If you want to swear you swear'. She said, 'Don't worry about anybody else, if you want to swear, you want to hit something, you hit something, but don't hit me'. She was trying to make it jokey for us.

> They were there if we needed them for a bit of support. They also made it not as traumatic as what it could have been 'cos they did have a laugh and a joke occasionally with us. They knew exactly sort of what the situation was. I think if they hadn't have been so sort of calm about it... sort of every so often they come in... I mean a couple of times they came in to give Peter a cuddle. Just to sort of say you know when they went off shift and everything... they sort of come in to say goodbye... I think we appreciated it a lot more. They were ever so good... everything we got up the hospital I think was ever so good.

Sue did not realise how difficult and traumatic it had all been until she began to discuss what had happened with her community midwife and GP who helped her to piece together her experience. She has been told her next baby will be delivered by caesarean section and is interpreting the stillbirth of her first baby as positively contributing to the safe delivery of her anticipated second baby. She does not feel bitter about her experience and is very positive about her hospital care apart from resenting the registrar who 'gawped' at her.

Judith, an unpleasant delivery: miscarriage

The unpleasantness of the infection Judith had contracted made the delivery of her baby particularly difficult. She was very tired and influenced by the diamorphine. The midwife asked the registrar to examine Judith only to discover that she was about to deliver. With hindsight the midwife wished she had delivered the baby herself, although since the registrar was there it was reasonable for him to continue. From Judith's point of view a stranger, who did not relate to her, delivered her baby:

> The registrar entered with a flurry like they do. He got all excited that the baby had started to move so as I say I knew it was on its way sort of thing. She pulled it. It was a tug-o'-war sort of thing. You know real brutishness... I could feel that it was out... It must have been stuck somewhere. And there was this awful smell, dreadful smell... it obviously was infected. The midwife pulled a blanket down so I couldn't see the baby straight away... I can't remember. I think the doctor took it out or something. When the doctor took it out the midwife said something like, 'Oh he's gone to look for some antibiotics', or something like that, there was a source of infection there. But I mean I was in tears at that time. It was the first time I cried there. Because I knew that was when the flood gates were going to open.

Labour and delivery

These women's experiences of labour and delivery are very different. Many factors – physical, psychological and social – will influence a woman's experience of labour but will include the gestation, the reason the pregnancy has gone wrong, the level of intervention necessary and her experience of pain, along with her own personal circumstances, psychological make-up and the support that she has. In addition some deliveries are clearly more unpleasant than others. Women's expectations, which will be based on their knowledge and experience of labour as well as what they have understood from the preparation they have, are also important.

The women will also be in the first phases of understanding that their baby has died or is dying with the powerful and confused feelings that this will arouse. They are likely to be at different stages in understanding and accepting this, as is illustrated above. They will also be concerned about what their baby will be like. It is likely they will have fears based in reality and in fantasy about what they will produce, associated with a sense of personal responsibility and failure.

Midwives are faced with the responsibility of helping women in this complex situation. In addition to the duties to assist and support women, common to the delivery of a live baby, the midwife is responsible for providing a high level of emotional support, preparing for the dead baby, facilitating grief and providing information so that the right decisions can be made. These women praised highly their skills in doing this:

> They were excellent, very caring and understanding. I didn't feel judged at all. I thought everyone understood why we were doing what we were doing and supported it really. They were medically and emotionally competent.
> Linda

> I simply could not fault them.
> Jenny

> Everyone did everything they could.
> Sheila

❏ The relationship between the midwives and women

> I don't think many of them after a while would remember what we did to them... but they will remember how they were treated and what the doctor said and how he said it, who was with her when it happened and the support that she got there.
> Midwife

The women's accounts of their labour and delivery confirm that the relationship a midwife is able to develop with a woman appears to be the basis of these women's experiences of good care. They had shared this deeply distressing, frightening and shocking experience with someone who connected with them, made them feel safe and appeared to feel comfortable with the experience themselves.

When a woman delivering a dead or dying baby is well cared for by a midwife a special relationship is established which can be characterised as an equal partnership. A deep and mutual respect appears to develop from the midwife for the woman's ability to bear the physical and emotional pain and from the woman for the midwife's skill in helping her, in being with her, in sharing and offering assistance and in her acceptance of what can be construed as unacceptable.

In turn the midwives described how important it was to form a trusting relationship with the woman:

> The secret is getting that rapport going really, where you can talk openly. I'm not frightened about talking about the problems that are going on as well. I think some people with death, whether it be with babies, adults or terminally ill people, they can't actually say, 'Isn't it terrible, your baby has died?' And I think sometimes that is called for, sometimes it's not. But I think to be able to be honest and open, it's very difficult for some people because they've still got that protective shell on.

Open discussion about how a woman is feeling and what she wants and is worried about is a feature of the relationship. Another midwife described her involvement with a woman as a 'constant struggle' to explore with her what was going to be right for her and a recognition that she had to work that out with her, that as the professional she did not necessarily know best.

Whilst the skill of the midwife in developing this relationship is crucial, it is a two-way process and there will be some women who are less able to participate in it. Mary described how, during her labour, pain relief was always too little and too late and how she felt completely alone and abandoned. In contrast her midwife described her as having all the pain relief available but as frightened of the pain and having a low pain threshold. The midwife reported that the unit was not very busy and she was available to be with the woman. In her view she was constantly popping in and out, which was substantiated in the notes. When interviewed six months after the stillbirth of her baby Mary described the midwifery staff as 'very good but pushed'. She was generally dissatisfied with her care but recognised that she did not want help that focused on her grief. Analysis of her case as a whole shows that none of the staff who cared for her and her partner managed to establish meaningful contact with her. Whilst actively seeking help from a range of professionals she frequently rejected the help that was offered.

It would appear that it is easier to establish a constructive relationship with the women who are more psychologically straightforward, emotionally open and communicative, not necessarily the most articulate or intelligent. Without the relationship it is much harder to provide effective care.

❏ Pain relief

> my leg was dead completely... you're only supposed to be numb from your belly button down. I was sort of numb all the way up. Every so often they would turn it off and that's when I'd sort of start feeling the pain again. I mean they ended up doubling the dose... I was as high as a kite basically... I mean I was just smiling, laughing, all sorts. Because of all the drugs I'd had.
>
> Sue

All the women whose labour was induced were given high doses of diamorphine. Those whose babies were stillborn were also given an epidural anaesthetic during labour. Two of the women whose pregnancies were terminated were also given an epidural anaesthetic for the removal of the remains of the placenta; the third had an ERPC under general anaesthetic.

The women had high expectations of pain relief. They said they had been told at diagnosis and once admitted to hospital that they 'need not suffer', they 'could have anything they wanted'. It was common for them to request caesarean section, which was refused, or to say, 'I want to be out of it.' Although one woman said the pain relief always came too late, contrasting with her midwife's view that 'she had double doses of everything', in general the women said that their frequent requests for pain relief were met with little delay. Midwives described discussion about and ensuring the availability of pain relief as an important part of their task. Anaesthetists saw the prompt delivery of their service as essential in these circumstances and their compassion and technical ability were appreciated by the women.

However, the high level of pain relief appears to create problems for some of the women. Whilst one of the women having a termination appreciated the pain relief the diamorphine brought, saying 'once it worked it was quite nice' (Linda), the others all commented on the debilitating consequences, saying they were 'drifting', 'out of it' or 'high as a kite' (Sue) and for one 'the pictures [on the wall] were at 45 degrees and crawling up the wall' (Judith). They said they did not know what was happening to them and were dependent on others afterwards to tell them.

There is clearly an ethos that a woman should suffer as little as possible, that requests for pain relief should be met, and perhaps a reluctance among some staff to challenge a woman's demands. One midwife described how the woman she was caring for had a 'low pain threshold' and was given an epidural 'when she truly wasn't in labour but because of her situation nobody could argue with her, nobody could say "no you can't" or "that's not a good idea"'. Another that she thought it was 'cruel to let someone go through as much pain as a woman in normal labour... We can give as much diamorphine as we like because we haven't got to think about the baby at that stage.' However, Jane described how she was helped by her mother, saying in early labour that she probably didn't need so much diamorphine yet and how her request for an early epidural was resisted, which in retrospect she appreciated.

In the past the lack of appropriate pain relief has been a feature of women's criticisms about their health care. It would clearly be wrong to deny women pain relief if it can help them but there is perhaps a reluctance to accept that the delivery of a dead or dying baby cannot be pain free. There will be emotional as well as physical pain. Pain relief cannot take away the emotional pain and in causing confusion may add an extra dimension to women's distress.

❏ The role of hospital doctors

Unless there was particular cause for concern the women had little contact with doctors during labour and delivery and they valued the respect that was shown for their privacy. A couple of the women also interpreted this as a demonstration of confidence in the skills of the midwives. When the consultant or registrar popped in to express his sympathy and availability if needed, the women appreciated and seemed to attach particular significance to this, out of all proportion to the time it must have taken. For one woman the consultant she briefly saw in hospital then became the person she wanted to see afterwards regardless of whether she was his patient or not. The women felt avoided if a senior doctor did not express his concern and always commented negatively on this.

Unusually, the consultant had an active role in the management of Jenny's care and was present for the delivery of her babies, which was important to her. The midwife valued his assistance generally but commented on the active support he, as a man, was able to give Jenny's husband, allowing her to concentrate on the delivery and handling of the babies.

The registrars were involved with the women largely when difficulties arose. They usually had little contact with the women beforehand. Judith's baby was delivered by a registrar unknown to her. Sue resented the intrusion of the registrar who came to see her during her long labour but did little:

> It was the way he came in several times and he just stared at us, ...didn't say nothing ...I don't know whether he couldn't handle it... He just stared at us. Sort of to say, 'There's nothing I can really do much.'

She later discussed with the registrar her request for a caesarean section, which was refused. The registrar was very concerned about her and unsure what more he could do to help:

> I always feel that I wish there was something that you could give them in the way of support. But I don't know whether that's possible really and I don't know, perhaps the doctor isn't the right person to become involved.

❑ Gaining consent for the post mortem

Gaining consent for the post mortem is a sensitive task. From the woman's point of view obtaining sufficient information in order to make the decision about the appropriateness of a post mortem, giving consent and agreeing to the research clause are separate activities but do not appear to have been treated as such. The women were approached for their consent either by a midwife or doctor, usually an SHO, and two of the women were approached by staff they had not met before. Four of the women objected to the research clause on the post mortem form and two reported that when they asked about this the staff said they were unaware that it was there or were unable to give the women adequate information.

Two of the women did not agree to the post mortem. Jenny did not think a post mortem was necessary as she knew why her babies had died and Sheila objected to a post mortem but agreed to blood and skin tests.

❏ Involving partners, family and friends

Apart from Lisa the women's partners were with them during their hospital admission. In addition friends and family visited the three women whose babies were stillborn. All the women reported that the hospital staff made their partner, family or friends very welcome. In Jane's words:

> The hospital were amazing... All they ever did was ask if we wanted more tea and give us more chairs... nobody seemed to raise an eyelid that there were so many people around.

The midwives clearly perceived caring for and involving women's partners as an important and sometimes difficult part of their role. They were aware that some of the partners found being present during labour and delivery difficult and that the women were, understandably, unable to focus on and sometimes unaware of their partner's needs. Several of the midwives commented on the support that doctors who were male were able to offer the women's partners if they were involved in the woman's care.

■ Hospital care: the baby

❏ Women's views on the handling of their baby

Table 4.6 summarises the contact the women had with their baby and their feelings about it. The women and their partners differed in the amount and nature of the contact they had with their babies but all were helped to do what was right for them. Six of the women were universally high in their praise for this aspect of their care. The midwives gave information, discussed the options with them and helped to prepare them accurately for their baby.

Two of the women were critical of this aspect of their care. Lisa, who was very distressed, was cared for on the emergency ward where staff are less experienced in delivery and the handling of a dead, immature fetus. She described the staff as being as helpful as they could but their lack of experience meant options were not discussed with her. The nurse disappeared in response to another patient's demands when she was about to deliver and she was told not to look at her baby when he was born, although she did see him later. She feared the baby was breathing and that this was being kept from her.

Mary, who was critical of many aspects of her care, was reluctant to see her baby. She objected to the baby being brought into the room completely covered with a quilt that was not removed until the Moses basket was placed on her lap and also, fearing the baby would deteriorate, to the baby being left in the room next door ready for them to see again if they wished. Her criticisms are perhaps a reflection of the difficulty she and her partner were having in facing the enormity of what had happened.

Table 4.6 Stillbirth, late miscarriage and termination: the baby

	Gestation (weeks)	Discussion of handling of the baby		Contact with the baby			Baby taken home	Family/ friends saw baby	Woman's feelings about seeing the baby		Mementoes		Women's description of disposal arrangements	Visit grave
		Before labour	During labour	Straight away	Later on delivery suite	Again in hospital			At the time	6 months later	Photo	Other		
Mary	36	✓	✓	–	✓	–	–	–	reluctant; felt pressured and refused to see again	traumatised by seeing the baby; regrets didn't see again	✓	✓	private burial	✓
Sue	41	✓	✓	–	✓	partner only	–	✓	reluctant; shocked by baby's appearance	very pleased she'd seen him	✓	–	hospital burial	✓
Jane	36	✓	✓	✓	✓	✓	✓	✓	'beautiful, perfect'	especially pleased baby had been at home with them	✓	✓	private cremation	✓
Jenny	23	✓	✓	✓	✓	✓	✓	✓	'normal thing to do'	wishes she could have spent more time at home with them	✓	✓	private cremation	✓
Judith	23	✓	✓	✓	–	–	–	–	said 'hallo and goodbye'; at peace	constantly regrets not seeing him again	✓	–	hospital funeral	–
Linda	21	–	✓	–	✓	–	–	–	limited contact; pleased but 'a bit gory'	no regrets	✓	✓	hospital disposal	–
Sheila	21	✓	✓	✓	✓	–	–	–	pleased	no regrets	✓	–	hospital burial	✓
Lisa	17	–	–	no because told not to look and baby was removed	✓	no because she didn't know this was possible	–	–	looked perfect except for black bits on head	no regrets	✓	–	hospital burial	✓

Six months after the birth none of these women, apart from Mary, had any regrets about the decisions they had made at the time. Although several women said they regretted they had not had more time with their baby this appeared to be more a reflection of the longing and searching for what they had lost than of the lack of opportunity that was created for them at the time. It is clear that the women were offered a very high standard of care.

❏ Jane's experience of being with her stillborn baby

I kept asking... the midwives... what she was going to look like rather than why. I was frightened I would hate her when I saw her.

When she was born the midwife held her up so I could see her. I didn't want to hold her at that point... I surprised myself... I didn't have any tears or anything, so that was great you know... Then Graham held her for a long time and cut the cord... And then they gave Lucy to me when I was ready and immediately he gave her to me I started feeling sick. Whether that was purely the drugs or whether it was psychological – I suspect it was a mixture... Then my mother came, then the rest of the family... I don't know what the time was by then.

[Later] I put her nappy on. It was such a compulsion, it was very intimate I suppose. I put her babygro on and Graham put her socks on.

The midwife took a hand and a footprint and a lock of her hair.

It was the first time I'd looked at her head because she'd had the hat on because of all the moulding and it didn't go back because she didn't have the muscles... She'd got black curly hair which was amazing because that's what I wanted her to have... [like her partner]... it made me feel very sad.

The couple moved from the delivery suite to the bereavement room on the postnatal ward where they spent the rest of the night sharing a double bed with Lucy, leaving the next morning:

We left hospital by the back entrance with Lucy and went home. Friends and family visited. It was so important that she had been in our home, we felt her presence... I have a vivid memory of coming down into the kitchen to see my sister-in-law cuddling Lucy next to my brother on the sofa reading the newspaper. What a good memory that is... It was important to see her deteriorate a bit... she was dead and you really had to take that on board.

It was a very hot day and they took Lucy back to the hospital earlier than they had anticipated. The next day they returned to the labour ward to see Lucy in the room where she was born:

> She was obviously very cold then and that was all right actually but again her skin was beginning to pucker a bit and she had perfect skin on her face and that was good because in a way we had decided that it was time to say goodbye and we had to do it. Much as I was saying I want to have her preserved so that I can see her every day... but you know that's unhealthy but that's how I was feeling.

The community midwife came in and saw her and held her which they found very helpful.

> Saying goodbye to her was the hardest thing but we had an hour on our own with her... I do understand other cultures like the Jewish culture where they wail... that's what we needed to do. But we were determined not to leave her in that kind of state so we spent a long time and leaving her was the most difficult thing. And we came back here [home] had a large gin and tonic and some friends cooked us a meal, which was wonderful.

❏ The implications of changing views

Fifteen years ago it is unlikely that Jane would have had the opportunity to be with her baby like this. Today professionals would be criticised for not making it possible if the parents wished. It is now generally accepted that seeing the baby is helpful to parents. This view is not based on research evidence that psychological damage is caused if the baby is not seen but on the understanding that knowing and saying goodbye to your baby facilitates grieving and that many women report that they want, need to and find it helpful, and if they do not, deeply regret it. Contact with the baby, even if it is dead, can be seen as part of the bonding process.

As with the birth of a live baby parents will differ in the amount and sort of contact they wish to have with their baby initially. However, unlike with the birth of a live baby, parents are limited in the time they can have with their baby and in addition are faced with the reality of their baby's death. This places responsibilities on staff to ensure parents know of and maximise the opportunities they have in the limited time available.

Opportunities that were initially created for parents whose babies were stillborn are now being extended to those whose babies are born before 24 weeks gestation as a result of either miscarriage or termination. Practice has changed considerably in recent years and is continuing to do so. Differences in professionals' ideas about what is acceptable are inevitable when professional practice is changing in response to a changing climate of opinion.

Individuals will have different exposure to the changes in practice and opportunities to develop their ideas may be limited. For example, one GP was shocked by the photographs a woman had of her babies delivered at 23 weeks gestation and thought it unusual to have them. A consultant thought the arrangements made for dressing a baby born at 23 weeks gestation and for the funeral were going too far. Another GP, whilst supportive of the opportunities a woman had to be with her baby, thought that she would have been unable to hold a dead baby like that and was concerned about the reactions of the person developing the photographs. A midwife was clearly worried that her colleagues would think that the encouragement she gave a woman to take her baby home was 'over the top'.

There is no suggestion that, for the health professionals caring for these women in the maternity unit, either their own views or what they thought their colleagues thought appropriate limited in any way the opportunities they were able to provide for these women. However, it cannot be ignored that providing the sort of care that Jane had challenges fundamental, commonly held ideas about life, death and acceptability, which imposes constraints on women, their partners and health professionals alike.

❏ Fears about the baby

> There is a slight concern in your mind that you might freak out, you know and start screaming... but I never cease to be amazed at the bravery of these women. Because I know that when I first came into this job... the thought of looking at a dead baby just horrified me... I remember... the first time that there was a dead baby here and I thought well I've got to go and look at it because I've got to get over this. And so I went into the sluice and looked at the baby and touched it but I admit that I was really frightened. And you know even four years down the road I'm just getting away with it.   Midwife

Although this midwife expressed her concerns more bluntly than most, she expressed fears that most people, professionals and parents alike, have about the reality of the relatively uncertain state of the dead baby that is to be born as well as the way everybody involved will react emotionally. Gestation, how long the baby has been dead, abnormality and the delivery will all affect the state of the baby but whatever the particular circumstances there is an underlying fear for all involved. Dead and abnormal babies and those of early gestation may inevitably and quite naturally arouse feelings of revulsion or fear of the potentially overwhelming nature of these feelings.

Individuals will differ in what they feel comfortable with and in what they consider acceptable. Since it is unlikely they will have given this much thought before and time is limited, the women and their partners are dependent on the professionals at the time to help them to contain their inevitable anxiety and make the most of the opportunities available to them. In order to provide this sort of care staff have to develop a degree of confidence themselves and be able to communicate this to their patients. Linda described the midwives caring for her as 'medically and emotionally competent, comfortable with handling the baby. It was not a problem to them.'

❑ Role of the midwives

Preparation by the midwife

The midwife has the sensitive task during labour of preparing a woman and her partner for the delivery of their baby; of enabling them to do what is right for them; of understanding how they might be feeling; of giving information, making appropriate suggestions and giving real choices; and of allowing time for them to make their own decisions. Although there may be a degree of uncertainty about the state of the baby on delivery, for example the extent of the abnormality or maceration, accurate information will help the midwife to answer any questions the mother may have. There may be concerns that the baby will breathe and anxieties about how this should be handled. It requires an openness on the part of the midwives and a willingness to share their own uncertainties. Jenny's midwife described how she prepared the couple for the birth of their babies, reassuring them and containing their anxiety:

> it had been explained [by the doctors] that the pregnancy was such an early gestation [23 weeks] that really the babies didn't actually stand a chance of surviving, although at that stage we couldn't say whether the babies would be stillborn or born alive. They were just too early... And I went on to discuss this at length both with her and her husband and of course they brought out many things. It was very very difficult, because it was 'What shall we do if the babies are born alive and we know that we can't do anything for them?'... The parents... how they... they kept on, 'How will we react? How will you react?'
>
> I said 'Well the choice, you know, it's absolutely your choice of what I do, when your babies are delivered.' And suggesting or putting ideas over, 'Would you like me to handle your babies, immediately they are delivered? Would you prefer me to wrap the babies up? Would you prefer me to leave the babies exactly as they are? Would you prefer...?' There are lots of options, making it very plain really that as time went on, if she decided at the last minute, 'I really don't want this, I've changed my mind', trying to make both of them feel that there were no hard and fast rules. It was really very very difficult, you know emotionally, for all of us really.

...At times they sort of wavered and sort of said, 'Oh I don't know whether we will be able to cope when the time comes.' ...So I said, 'When the time comes we will just take it step by step and see how you feel then... You really cannot foretell how you are going to react because you haven't been through the experience before.'

The midwife helped the couple focus on their babies and enabled them to start the grieving process. This couple were emotionally open and ready to communicate with her in this way. Once their babies were born they spent a lot of time with them. Other couples were less receptive and more reluctant.

Helping parents to be with their baby: Linda

Some of the women saw their baby straight away whilst others had agreed to the midwife washing and wrapping the baby for them to see later when they felt ready. The midwife has an important role in helping parents to spend time with their baby. It is a delicate balance of reassuring and encouraging, of being there and of allowing parents time on their own. Linda's pregnancy was terminated because of her baby's severe abnormalities. Her baby was given to her straight away wrapped in the blanket the couple had brought for him. The midwife describes how she helped the couple be with their baby:

Her husband was there but he wasn't quite sure what he wanted to do about the birth of the baby... And he wasn't able to cope initially so he went out and Linda and I sat together with the baby and she held the baby, and we looked at it together. And it had obvious abnormalities, externally as well. And my policy usually is to not say anything, just quietly be supportive and let her look at the baby, which she did do. And then she pointed out that the baby had a cleft lip and palate as well. And I said, 'Yes I noticed but I just wanted you to have time to adjust to it yourself.' And really I think that was a big relief to her because she had made a really difficult decision and she hadn't really known whether it was the right one. And to see that the baby would have had to have a lot of surgery for that as well, I think it really relieved her a great deal. So I stayed with her for about 25 minutes and we looked at the baby and we talked and then I left her alone with the baby for a while.

Then I went and found her husband. And he had sort of gone off to sort of recover himself really. He was a lovely man, but you know, he was a typical English man, in that emotions are very much tucked inside and he didn't cope brilliantly. But I took him into a room on his own. And we talked about whether he would like to see the baby and

I explained that there were other abnormalities. And then he decided that he would go in and be with Linda, which was nice... And he did very well I think. He actually cried quite a lot, which is often a pattern actually. The man cries whilst the ladies go through everything.

The time they had together with their baby became a focus for their grief. They gave him the name they had chosen for him. Linda described a feeling of being at peace and of having said goodbye to her baby and at that point she felt she did not need to see the baby again. Six months later she regretted that she had not had more time with him.

When parents are reluctant to see the baby: Sue

Most parents will fear what their baby will look like and how they will react. Some will find the idea of a dead baby deeply abhorrent and will be very reluctant to see their baby but, if they do not, may regret it later. Sue was horrified at the prospect of seeing her baby. Her baby was stillborn at term but the delivery had been difficult. The midwife described the baby as 'awful looking'. Sue discussed it with the midwife:

> She said, 'Whatever you want I'll do it'. She said, 'You can have the baby and see it' and Peter said, 'No I couldn't do that.' And I couldn't do that. I said what I want is if you can take it away. She says, 'I'll wrap it myself and take it away, wash it, clean it, dress it in a babygro', because we actually gave a babygro for it... 'and put it in the baby basket'. And then she said, 'you can see it straight away if you want', but, knowing what we've been through, up till half past two, quarter to three sort of thing and I'm absolutely gazonked and Peter was, so we didn't see it till the next morning. She brought it in about ten o'clock...

> It was a lot worse than I thought it would be. I mean they said it would be like a baby asleep but where it sort of got the blood around its lips, where it was bruised... it was a little bit discoloured as well because of what had gone on [difficult delivery]... And she brought the Moses basket and put it on the bed. We had a look and it was a bit of a shock. But if I hadn't have seen it, I don't think I'd be able to cope as well... she did say sort of there might be a little bit of blood around the lips... And she took the baby away and put it in a room. It was the room next door. So if we wanted to go and see it we could... Peter went to say goodbye before we left the hospital. I couldn't do that, 'cos it was hard enough for me to see the baby as it was...

The midwife described how reluctant the couple were. At the delivery they wanted the baby taken straight away and then kept putting off seeing him. They were eventually with him for about ten minutes. Sue did not pick up her baby nor did she see him a second time. Six months later she acknowledged how difficult it had been to see him but was very pleased she had. She had no regrets about not seeing him again.

Sue did not feel pressured into seeing her baby although the midwife felt she had to persuade her. Mary did feel pressured into seeing her baby and was shocked at having to do so. She described seeing the baby as traumatising and refused to see her baby a second time. Six months later her biggest regret was that she had not done so. In these situations the midwife is in a powerful position to influence the decision the woman makes. A midwife describes the difficulty in helping a woman to decide to see her baby or not:

> You are saying to a woman whether or not to see her baby, whether or not you persuade her... you are in a very privileged position... sometimes it's very difficult, especially if you've got a baby that's very disfigured and has been dead a long time... They don't know whether they want to see the baby and also fetuses don't look like babies as we imagine... they are expecting to see a baby as a term baby only smaller and it can be a shock.

> each person is an individual and although the ideal is yes they should all have the opportunity to see the baby and say goodbye and finish off... it isn't always appropriate. I had a lady... if she had seen the baby she would have had nightmares about it forever. The baby didn't look very nice and... she was a lady who said to me 'if it looks nice I'll see the baby' and it took me a long time to talk to her and say well you know, the baby had been dead about a week. And on that occasion we didn't see the baby together and I feel that it was the right decision... So I do work towards that goal [of seeing the baby] but I'm not rigorous about it.

This midwife was skilled in creating the opportunity for a woman to see her baby if she wished, in helping her make the decision that was right for her. Clumsily insisting a woman sees her baby against her will is a modern form of bullying as oppressive as whisking the baby out of sight, as was done in the past.

When the baby is abnormal: Sheila

Individuals, however, react differently. Assumptions cannot be made about gestation or the degree of abnormality affecting parents' wishes to see or be with their baby. Sheila's baby had an abnormality incompatible with life. She was very philosophical about her baby:

It's one of these things. These things do happen. You've just got to learn to live with it ain't ya? I mean, I know he's dead but he's not forgotten, but my life still has to go on, same as Kevin's, you know? But it ain't stopped us from trying again...

They actually said to me when he was born, 'Do you want us to wash him or take him straight away' but I wanted to hold him then – 'cos Kevin was there when I had him as well. That's what they did. The midwife took him away, washed him, they dressed him up and they brought him back to us. And we held him. And we were there – all day Saturday with him. And then Saturday night we went down to a – they call it a bereavement room, me and Kevin. And then they put him in the morgue then at the hospital... I mean I still have to carry him didn't I?... I mean even though he's dead there is still that bond there, if you know what I mean, like he was if he was alive... I think that was long enough – for both of us really. They even said to me – one of the other midwives who had come on the day shift – she says to me, 'Do you want to see him on the Sunday before you go in the morning?' I went, 'No, I've seen him, I've held him and that's enough now.' ...His [Kevin's] dad came up on Saturday when the baby was still in the room. So he see him and that and it seems funny but we were speaking to him even though he was dead, we were still speaking to him.

The consultant described the baby as 'a mermaid with fins... every woman's nightmare' and thought Sheila would have found the baby repulsive. At the delivery Sheila had only seen her baby swathed in a blanket but clearly felt comfortable cuddling and being with him. At her follow-up appointment she spotted the slides in her medical notes. She asked to see them and persisted when the consultant attempted to dissuade her. She said she wanted to know and was not outwardly distressed. A photograph of her baby, her first son, is in pride of place on top of the TV. Six months after the birth she had no regrets. The couple made arrangements for the burial of their baby and Sheila's partner regularly visits the grave.

❑ Seeing the baby again

Opportunities for seeing the baby again

All the women who were cared for on the delivery suite were offered as much opportunity to be with their baby as they wished. The flexible and sensitive approach of the midwives enabled them to do so. The contact the women had with their babies varied from viewing for ten minutes sometime after delivery (Sue) to continuous contact throughout the hospital stay and taking the baby home (Jane).

Mary and Sue saw their babies briefly on the delivery suite whilst Judith and Linda spent longer with their babies. None of these women wanted to see their baby again. In contrast Jane, Jenny and Sheila had their babies with them all day or overnight. Jane and Jenny returned after their discharge to see their babies again in the hospital. Sheila did not see her baby again as she had mistakenly understood she would have to go to the mortuary to do so. This was not suggested to her and arrangements would willingly have been made for the baby to be returned to the ward, as is the normal practice.

Creating opportunities for the women to see their baby in the hours or days after delivery means that appropriate arrangements have to be made for the storage of the baby's body. If the parents did not want the baby with them in the immediate hours after delivery, the baby was kept in a nearby room. If a room had been unavailable the sluice would have been used. Ultimately, the baby was removed to the mortuary. When the parents were seeing the baby some time after the delivery likely changes in the state of the baby's body were sensitively explained to them. Jane commented on how helpful this was as part of the process of recognising her baby's death.

Jane took her baby home with her from hospital (see above) whilst Jenny's babies were brought to her house prior to the funeral. She would have liked to have had longer with her babies at home but understood that the babies' bodies could only be released to the funeral directors. Jenny was not aware that this is not the legally the case. Both of these women described how being able to take their baby home was the most important part of the contact they had with their baby. It secured in their mind the existence of their baby as part of their normal lives and provided memories of the baby that were a source of future comfort.

Lisa's concern about the whereabouts of her baby

It is common for women to worry about what will happen to their baby once it has been taken away. Although this was of concern to most of the women it was acutely troubling to Lisa, who regretted her decision to have a termination and was critical of the handling of her baby post-delivery. She describes her feelings of being empty and alone and her concerns about the whereabouts of her baby's body:

> I vividly remember saying, 'I don't want my baby down in the mortuary, it's cold.' And she said, 'Well we wrapped it up.' It's just the thought of it laying down there on it's own. I knew it wasn't alive, that it couldn't feel it, it couldn't feel being cold. But it's my baby and I wouldn't treat my baby like that.

> I just wanted to be with it where it should have been. It shouldn't have been there. It shouldn't have been laying on a cold piece of whatever it lays on in the fridge, it should have been with me. And it was all taken

away. I've been through that and I've got nothing. But I would have, I really would have you know, I would have walked out. I would have walked out of hospital with it at one point. I was going to get out of bed and I was going to find the mortuary. I wanted to go and get it back...

No, you're there in this room with nothing. And you know there was something there, you know you're bleeding and you know, you can still feel that you've just had [a baby] but you've got nothing to hold and nothing to look at... with all the others, even the first night after you've had them you wake up to look to see if they're all right. I was doing all those things and there was nothing to look at. It was just empty. The whole place was just empty. There was nothing. I could have been the only person in the world then. There was no-one and nothing else there.

Her inner turmoil is perhaps a reflection of the lack of acceptance of the decision she had made along with the relative inexperience of the staff on the emergency unit in labour and delivery. The nurses caring for Lisa had sought advice from the midwives and bereavement officer and had discussed with Lisa the options in her care.

❏ Photographs and mementoes

The current practice of providing photographs and mementoes of the baby was valued by these women. They all had photographs of their baby and some had other mementoes – hand and footprints, a lock of hair – as well. For some of the women they assumed a greater importance than others but six months after the birth none regretted having them. Jane and Sue were dependent on the photographs that were taken at the time to help them to understand what had happened and what they had been through as well as confirming the reality of their baby. Jenny valued the photographs, which she framed and displayed in her home. Although Judith had seen and held her baby her memories were also based on how she thought her baby would have been as much as the reality. Several months later she wrote:

At the time of my miscarriage we were offered a photograph of the baby which we did not want. I knew it was in the notes so I asked for it at my outpatient appointment. I was disappointed in the photo. The baby was wrapped in a blanket with only the head showing. I would have preferred to be able to see all my baby in the photo as it was her hands and feet with fingernails that I was amazed at and remember. I don't really know if I do want the photo but it is nice to know it is in the bottom of the drawer with hand and feetprints and weight recorded.

❏ **Disposal arrangements**

All the women who were cared for on the maternity unit said they were able to make the arrangements for the disposal of their baby's body that was right for them and that the staff involved – the midwives and the registration officer – sensitively helped them to do this. The options were explained to them and time was given for decisions to be made. They made different choices for burial or cremation, for the hospital to make the arrangements or to do it themselves, and how public to make the ceremony if they had one (see Table 4.6).

Neither Linda or Judith, whose babies were terminated owing to abnormality, wished to be involved in the disposal arrangements for their baby or to attend a ceremony of any kind. They wanted the hospital to take the responsibility. They made their decision following discussions with midwifery staff and the bereavement officer. The staff and women referred to the cremation of their baby. The baby would have been incinerated by the hospital.

Regardless of the gestation of their baby or the reason for the death, all the other women arranged burial or cremation, either themselves or through the hospital, and were helped to do so. Several of the parents described how helpful the existence of the grave or plaque was in the coming months and visited it regularly.

Lisa, who was cared for on the emergency ward, was critical of the muddled information she was given on different occasions and by different people about the arrangements she could make for the disposal of her baby's body and that she was incorrectly told at one point that her baby had been disposed of. The complaint she made to the hospital was treated sensitively and appropriately and she was helped to make the arrangements for a hospital funeral, which she attended.

■ **Hospital care: management post-delivery**

❏ **Staying on the delivery suite**

Three of the women transferred to the bereavement room prior to discharge. The others, who were not always offered the facilities of the bereavement room, were desperate to get home to be with other children or to their own bed or to get away from the hospital and the painful reality of the proximity of other successful mothers with healthy babies. Sue describes how she felt:

> I could have stayed longer. I think I was all right in myself but I think if I'd stayed any longer I think I would have ended up cracking up in the end. And I think you really want to come home and do your own thing. I was ready to come home... I think we needed our own bed and our own good night's sleep... Well, it was on the labour ward and

you've got all the... other people having babies and they've done well. I mean, every time sort of in between hearing them going through their pain you hear a baby cry. I think that would have done me in if I'd stayed any longer. I mean I got used to it, the two days I was up there. And I've got used to sort of seeing newborn babies now, people walking round with children. But it's going to be a bit hard for a while.

Mary, who remained on the delivery suite for ten hours after the birth, hated it, did not feel she belonged there and would have preferred to have been moved. She wanted to get home as soon as possible. Six months later she thought she had left hospital too soon.

❏ The bereavement room

Sheila and Jane valued the facilities that were offered: a double bed, the opportunity to be somewhere private with their partner, with their baby if they wished, and to sleep. Sheila described it as a 'real treat, it was home from home if you know what I mean. It didn't actually feel like you were in the hospital in that room.' However, it appears a difficult transition to make from the delivery suite, which has become a place of security, to somewhere new, where staffing levels are lower and contact with the staff often infrequent, at a time when the women are feeling particularly vulnerable. It is their first experience of facing the wider world. Jane describes her experience:

I got washed and taken down to a double bed on the postnatal ward at about five in the morning. I would have done anything at that stage. I was ambivalent about that because I wanted to stay on the labour ward and I wanted to stay in that room, because that's where I'd been for the last 48 hours and that was my life and I found it hard to get out of the room even. But it wasn't... they got me into bed and Graham got into bed and they lay Lucy [baby] between us. And that was lovely and then I went to sleep – I think Graham said I was unconscious almost before my head hit the pillow I was so tired. And I think we both woke up at about eight o'clock in the morning and there she was lying there and that was a bit difficult.

Judith described her experience of the bereavement room as a 'disaster'. The delivery of her baby had been made particularly unpleasant by the infection she had contracted. The contrast between how she was feeling and the smart decor were incongruous. Combined with what to her seemed like neglectful care she felt overwhelmed and abandoned:

Going down to that room was awful. The difference in care down there was what I feared. It was dreadful... We went downstairs into a beautifully carpeted room, an absolutely stark contrast... Up on the labour wards, you know, it's all out in the open, you know, it all happens, blood on the floor. And you go downstairs into this carpeted room, you know, don't get it dirty, brush it all under the carpet... It was a completely different attitude... The first thing I was greeted with was... the bed hadn't been made into a double bed. It was still a single. You know, nothing had been done to it. There was absolutely nothing there, like tissues or sanitary towels or anything that you might want...The midwife said to me, 'Oh come and go as you please. Come and go as you please, here's the key to the door and if you forget the antibiotics at four just give us a ring' and that was it. They waltzed off and we were stuck in this room... That room would have been all right if someone had just come in and explained. You know, just the normal procedure of welcoming someone to the ward really. I can understand their reasons, the midwives looking after women in bed with new babies... with live ones... Well I hated it there and I just wanted to go home.

Her distress was recognised and the doctor on duty offered to transfer her to the emergency ward, which she refused.

❑ Discharge from hospital

However desperate the women were to get home, leaving hospital was a big step, the first step in resuming life in an altered state without their baby yet no longer pregnant. To a greater or lesser extent all the women except Lisa formed a strong and intimate relationship with the midwife or midwives caring for them. On discharge from hospital not only do they normally leave their baby behind but they also leave the security of the institution and the relationships they had established there for the perhaps more uncertain terrain of family, friends and the community services.

None of the women reported feeling that they were in the way or that they were rushed by the staff to go home before they felt ready to. The women said they were given the information they needed, although they may not have been receptive to it, and on the whole their discharge from hospital was managed well. Sue was critical of the fact that she left hospital without the pain relief she needed and which was difficult to obtain once home. Judith was given conflicting information about when she could go home, which compounded her distrust of the staff on the postnatal ward. The women always appreciated the midwife who had cared for them coming to say goodbye.

■ Care after discharge from hospital

❑ Introduction

Difficulties in providing effective care after discharge from hospital: Jane's experience

Jane had excellent continuity of care. By chance her community midwife was on duty during her hospital admission and delivered her baby. She visited Jane frequently along with her colleagues in the three weeks post-delivery and played a crucial role in enabling the couple to talk about the death of their baby as well as offering more routine postnatal midwifery care. Although Jane has kept in touch with her community midwife, the regular visits inevitably ended, much to her regret. The community midwife arranged for the health visitor to visit, which Jane valued but she was unsure what was being offered and did not see her again. Her GP visited shortly after her discharge from hospital and Jane attended for a six week postnatal check. Around this time her consultant also visited her at home. Jane had agreed to a hospital support group contact but only saw her once. She approached SANDS, attended some of the meetings and was regularly in touch with her SANDS contact. She had a supportive partner and her friends, one in particular who had also had a baby who died, were helpful to her.

On the face of it Jane was offered much professional help but a more detailed examination of her experience reveals the discrepancy in meeting her needs. She continued to need to talk about the detail of what had happened but once the immediate postnatal period was over and the phase of active help had ceased, it was hard to know who to turn to. Nine weeks after her baby was stillborn she wrote:

> I have asked the hospital for my labour notes and Lucy's post mortem report. I received an acknowledgement but nothing since. I would like to go through all the information and my notes with one of the professionals involved. I do not disbelieve the information I have received but I need to see it all in black and white. I will then trust that no-one is trying to protect me. But who should I ask? I feel that the consultant and GP are not approachable enough and may get defensive about a request like this. The midwife who is my contact from the hospital support group visited once at home and seemed very ill at ease outside her professional domain. I have not contacted the health visitor since her initial visit. I found her great but I am not sure what she was offering. Would she be the appropriate person? The only other person I have considered is the community midwife [who delivered Lucy]. We have not seen each other but left a number of messages on answerphones! I think she is the person who I would like to ask to go through my notes as I feel that she has always been

honest and has genuinely given of herself. But, I'm not sure that this would be acceptable.

All in all, I don't seem to know what roles the professionals play – if any. I think that this is a problem as I would like to have someone contacting me monthly rather than having to do it all myself but perhaps that's me trying to shirk responsibility. Whereas, I think this explains part of it but also I feel that I have been in a fairly helpless emotional state, which prevents me seeking help. Perhaps this is why I write such lengthy accounts to you each month.

Jane needed ongoing professional support once the flurry of professional activity in the immediate period post-discharge was over but she was unable to ask for it and wanted to see the person she had become closest to, the community midwife. Obtaining Jane's notes was straightforward and she found it helpful but this did not resolve the problem of her need for ongoing help. About three months after the stillbirth she felt particularly low and abandoned and arranged to see a counsellor. She opted to make the arrangements privately rather than see the practice counsellor as she did not want it entered on her medical notes.

Women's differing needs: Sheila's experience

Women will differ in the definition of their needs, in their ideas about the acceptability of seeking help and in their expectations of it. Unlike Jane, who recognised that she accepted any form of help offered to her, Sheila lay at the opposite extreme and did not want to share her experience beyond her immediate family. Whilst it may be considered more acceptable to talk about stillbirth than termination Sheila's attitudes were more to do with her disinclination to turn to outsiders, whether they be lay or professional. She described her feelings shortly after her discharge from hospital:

I says at the moment I don't feel like really I need to go and talk to anybody about it... I mean I'm not hard myself but at the moment I don't need to... Before, me and Kevin we can sort these things out. I mean all my family is there for me. I can go down and spend as much time as I want with them at both their places. I mean she [sister] come up this week and stay with me as well. There's the dog and that. So I got all them round me.

Sheila's views did not change. She valued her appointment with her consultant, which she saw as having a very clear purpose, and saw her GP briefly for a sick note but did not see the need for further professional involvement.

Sources of help

In practice it is likely that women will get help from a variety of different sources. The quality of resources available to women will vary and they will make use of services in different ways. Some tasks clearly fall within a specific professional domain; for example, information about the results of tests and discussion about the reason for stillbirth, miscarriage or abnormality are the obstetrician's responsibility. Others, like the need for support and the opportunity to talk about what has happened, can potentially be met from a variety of lay and professional sources.

Table 4.7 summarises the help these women received and their evaluation of it. For five of the women one professional (a consultant, GP or community midwife) assumed a particular significance after their discharge from hospital. The women had mostly, prior to or during their hospital admission, established relationships with the people they considered helpful. A relationship based on trust, respect and understanding then developed. To a limited extent the women chose whom they wanted to help them and disregarded the professionals, who appeared less approachable, were less involved or uncomfortable with the experience. When needed the doctors were able to offer ongoing help to these women whereas the help the community midwives offered was time-limited.

Three of the women did not have a relationship with a 'significant professional'. Sheila clearly did not want professional help but Judith and Linda would have valued closer involvement with the community services. All three had pregnancies terminated because of abnormality and had relatively little contact with the community professionals prior to the termination. In turn, because the pregnancies were under 24 weeks gestation and perhaps considered less significant than later losses, combined with a sensitivity about termination and a desire not to intrude on an individual's personal decision, the professionals appeared ambivalent about offering help.

In comparison to the women whose babies were stillborn, who were routinely visited by their GP and community midwife, the women who miscarried or whose pregnancies were terminated because of abnormality were either asked if they wanted the community services involved or told of their availability and that it was up to them to make contact. Invariably, the women felt unable to do so and interpreted the lack of routine contact self-punitively, as a judgement on their actions. Linda's wishes about immediate follow-up care had been misinterpreted and she was concerned that no-one had contacted her:

> it just makes me feel .. that because I haven't got a baby it doesn't
> matter... Also I spoke to my GP. I did phone him myself... He'd been
> away... And normally he's very sweet and very caring so that was why
> I felt I wanted to phone him. And I thought he would visit but he
> didn't visit... He asked how I was, but he wasn't concerned about

Table 4.7 Stillbirth, late miscarriage and termination: women's perceptions of professional care and support from voluntary organisations in the six months following discharge from hospital

| | Hospital | | Significant person in aftercare | Primary care | | | Hospital support group | Self-help group | Professional help | Self-referral |
	Consultant follow-up	Genetic counsellor		GP	CMW	HV				
Mary	5/1	–	–	4	4	–	3 T/C only	4	bereavement counsellor 4 CPN 3	Natural health centre, healer
Sue	1	–	GP/CMW	1	1	–	2 T/C only		–	–
Jane	2	–	CMW	4	1	2		1	refused offer of practice counsellor	private counsellor
Jenny	1	–	GP	1	4	3 T/C only	3 T/C only	3 T/C only	CPN 3	–
Judith	2	1	–	4	4	–	3 T/C only	3 T/C only	–	–
Linda	1	–	–	2	5	–	4	1	–	–
Sheila	1	2	–	–	–	–	–	–	–	–
Lisa	–	–	GP	1	–	5	–	–	considering referral for counselling	–

1 = very helpful
2 = helpful with reservations
3 = neither helpful nor unhelpful
4 = unhelpful
5 = very unhelpful
T/C = telephone call
CMW = community midwife
CPN = community psychiatric nurse
HV = health visitor

seeing me… He did know what was going on. He had dictated a letter to be sent… When I had [my son] the GP came round and obviously I had the normal sort of ten days visits from midwives. Whereas, you know, this time there's sort of been nothing… And when I spoke to the community midwives this morning they said they don't normally visit… I feel it's because we made that decision, you know, there hasn't been any follow-up on us. I do feel that that is very bad. I'm not saying that they should visit for the ten days. I don't feel too bad… it's just different things… things like my milk's come in and obviously that's very painful.

They made it sound as if it was normal practice… Whether it's because people don't know how to react to you because of what we've done. Whether their beliefs are different and they feel that this is something we shouldn't have done. But then as a professional you know you should be able to deal with that and you shouldn't judge people in that sense.

Many of the women, regardless of the reason for their loss, were acutely sensitive to the reactions of others, thinking that professionals would not want to see them because they had no baby or because, like Linda, they would be judged for the decision they had made. Linda felt hurt and rejected by what she considered professional indifference. It was not intended: the professionals concerned viewed her as a coping, competent person with supportive family and friends, who would ask for help if she needed it. In the psychologically vulnerable period after the loss of a pregnancy it is extremely hard for women, however competent, to reach out for help. In addition professional help freely given acknowledges the importance of the baby and legitimates the loss.

❏ Hospital follow-up: the consultant appointment

All the women cared for in the maternity unit were offered and accepted follow-up appointments with their consultant which, apart from in one case (Mary), they described positively. Issues to do with the recent and future pregnancies were addressed and the results of the post mortem or any tests discussed. The women valued the access to the professional expertise of the consultants, who gave clear information in a straightforward way, answered questions honestly and did not dodge the difficult issues, gave their time and expressed their concern. When photos were given it was done sensitively and appropriately.

The appointments normally took place in the hospital, although Jane's consultant visited her at home. She said she did not like consultants much and felt 'a bit patronised' but appreciated the concern and the effort that was made to do a home visit, which helped to put her and her partner in a stronger position and enabled them to be more articulate.

Six months after her termination Lisa had not met with her consultant. She had a routine appointment (for her gynaecological condition) with her consultant one week after the termination, which she felt unable to keep as she was so distressed. Other appointments had been offered which she also failed to keep. Her GP had to ring the hospital for the results of the post mortem; Lisa would have liked her consultant to write to her.

For many women the follow-up appointment, normally at six weeks, becomes a milestone in the immediate period after their loss when questions will be answered and information gained. Judith and Linda were concerned about the delays in the follow-up appointment. Both were anxious for any available information as they wished to become pregnant again. Judith resented having to chase up her outpatient appointment and wrote:

> I asked my hospital contact to phone, I phoned and my GP phoned. I received it four weeks after leaving hospital. It was meant to be a six weeks appointment and it is in fact nearly nine weeks. I know it is only quibbling over a few weeks but it's surprising how you need something to latch onto and I wanted to know when my appointment was so I would know the date when I would get some feedback.

Linda waited nine weeks after her termination for her follow-up appointment. There was an administrative mix up because she changed consultants. During this time she imagined the baby to have been normal and the termination unnecessary. The post mortem revealed gross abnormality, confirming that she had made the right decision. The anguish this caused could have been avoided if she had been asked which consultant she wished to see and the appointment promptly arranged.

❏ The implications of worries about the cause of a stillbirth

A lack of explanation for the reason for a stillbirth is common. It is often the basis of anxiety for parents and professionals alike and colours the interactions that take place between women and their professional carers. The failure of professionals to deal with their own feelings can get in the way of their ability to offer effective help.

Jane and her partner were well informed and were able to accept that there was no definable cause for their baby's death. She commented that she thought her consultant was clearly relieved when she and her partner acknowledged this, which made the rest of their discussion easier. It was more difficult with her GP, whom she thought felt responsible in some way. She wrote:

I think I understand what it is like for her. She seemed very concerned that something had been missed during my pregnancy. I realised that she was having problems accepting what seemed like a completely normal pregnancy should end with a stillbirth. During my appointment I found myself reassuring her that I did not blame the medical profession for anything.

Mary and her partner found the lack of explanation for their baby's death hard to accept. They found the follow-up appointment with the consultant actively unhelpful and described the consultant as uninterested in them, irresponsible in not leading the discussion and irritated with their questions. The couple thought the consultant was defensive when they questioned the GP's role; the consultant found it difficult to answer their questions, not wanting 'to land other professionals in it' but also not wanting to 'blindly stick together and close ranks'. It was his view that nothing had been missed. The consultant offered them 'whatever they wanted next time'; they thought he had no specialist advice and could not be bothered. The consultant had made considerable effort to see them quickly at the end of a day's work; they thought he was ill prepared and too tired to see them. The woman reported that the consultant had said she would be neurotic in the next pregnancy, which was interpreted as an insult and a suggestion that she would go mad, although she was very concerned about her health; the consultant thought he was allowing her to make demands.

The consultant acknowledged that he hated follow-up interviews and those where 'you have to carry the can for others' made him cross. He was surprised at their response and thought they would be pleased that no abnormality had been detected. He realised he was the focus for their anger but criticised the couple as 'dumb and stupid' and was left feeling he could do nothing right. The couple were experienced as a 'bit odd' or 'difficult' by most of the professionals they encountered, were critical of their care and rejected a lot of the help that was offered to them. However, they later saw another consultant, who had expressed his sympathy to them in hospital after the delivery and who had impressed them as competent and reassuring. Given the choice at the time they would have asked to see him. They have been able to accept his help and six months after the stillbirth identified him as 'remaining a good source of support'. Mary feels he will always make time to talk to her, is really interested, has answered her questions, has talked about the next pregnancy and has taken her concerns about her physical ill-health seriously.

❑ GP follow-up

Offering effective long-term support

GPs are in a unique position to provide ongoing help to women as it is needed in the weeks and months after discharge from hospital. Three of the women received excellent care from their GPs, all of whom took responsibility for initiating and maintaining contact with the women. Jenny, who had a difficult pregnancy, valued highly the antenatal care and postnatal support from her GP. She initially saw him weekly and then fortnightly. Six months after the loss of her babies she continued to see him monthly. He has always suggested she make an appointment for the next week instead of letting her decide so that she can feel she is keeping in touch without wasting his time. Sue saw two of the GPs at her practice frequently in the weeks after the stillbirth. She felt she could contact them whenever she needed to and appreciated their support, the detailed information they gave about the traumatic delivery and the continued medical help for the infections she had. Both these GPs were concerned that they were 'feeling their way' and had not offered enough.

Apart from her parents, her GP is the only person Lisa talks to about the termination of her pregnancy, which she regrets and is deeply troubled by. She had discussed with him the decision about the termination prior to her admission to hospital and he phoned her after her discharge. The GP thought Lisa was treated badly by the system and that her feelings were perfectly legitimate in the circumstances. Whilst recognising the limitations of his counselling skills he was also concerned that Lisa would not accept help from anyone else and expressed concern as to who to refer her to if it became necessary.

To begin with she saw him twice weekly and wrote:

> We talked. I was also given tranquillisers... He listened. It was nice that he contacted me... Talking to him has become easier. He doesn't tell me what he thinks I want to hear... He seems to understand better than some women. He told me it was OK to have the feelings I had and encouraged me to write things down.

Two months later she wrote:

> I speak to him once a week or so. We use this time to go over anything that has happened since I last saw him. The appointments are always helpful, just because he listens... It's left open for me to chat any time... He lets me say and feel whatever I need without feeling silly. It's especially helpful to me as I feel unable to speak about it to most people.

Six months after the termination Lisa was surprised by the lack of progress she had made and described herself as 'going backwards'. She was considering the GP's suggestion to seek counselling help.

Rejecting the help that is offered

Jane and Mary, for different reasons, could not accept the help that was offered from their GP. Jane described her GP as awkward with emotional issues and said she did not feel comfortable talking with her:

> When I got home from hospital she visited on spec which was nice except she wanted to talk about my next pregnancy which I feel is a bit much. You know she said all the right things, she looked at the picture of Lucy but...

Jane's GP defined her role as clinical management but also wanted to express her sympathy and smooth the path for future medical care. Her GP also gave her the name of the counsellor at the surgery. She saw her GP again for the six week postnatal check, which she found helpful in confirming that she was physically well but felt the GP was finding it difficult to accept the stillbirth.

As with other aspects of her care Mary and her partner were critical of the care offered by the GP and, a couple of months after the stillbirth, changed to another practice. They questioned the GP's part in Mary's antenatal care, although there were no medical grounds for this. They were also upset by the lack of continuity of care provided by locum doctors at night. Mary had started to feel she was a nuisance and was not reassured about her concerns about her physical health. The GP saw her frequently after the stillbirth to offer her support as well as to address the concerns about her physical ill-health. The GP identified 'facilitating their grief' as a major task but one for which she did not feel well prepared and was aware that she was also 'picking up the pieces' from the hospital care, dealing with the anger and resentment the couple expressed about the other health professionals involved in their care.

Termination for abnormality

For different reasons the women whose pregnancy was terminated because of abnormality had little to do with their GP after the termination. In contrast to the GPs for the women whose babies were stillborn these GPs appeared ambivalent about their role, unsure of what to offer and expected the women to ask for help if they needed it. The sensitivities around termi- nation and the fact that GP care is not accepted as routine appear to get in the way of women getting the help they need.

Judith needed more help than she got but nevertheless appreciated the 'courtesy visit' made to her at home by a GP she hardly knew, who acknowledged she 'was in the wars having had three miscarriages'. He was the first person to recognise the cumulative impact of the termination and earlier miscarriages. He also gave her the information he had received from the hospital, which gave details of the infection that had probably contributed to the problems with her pregnancy.

Like the other women who had little regular contact with their GP after this first meeting Judith did not discuss her pregnancy directly or her feelings about it although she would have liked to, but needed to see her GP to obtain sickness certificates. She also consulted him about minor physical ailments. She became concerned that she would have an ectopic pregnancy and consulted her GP about a worrying pain in her side when she ovulated. She was reassured and was aware that her worries surfaced at the time her baby was due, when she felt very low.

Similarly, Sheila and Linda had little contact with their GP. This was unproblematic for Sheila. Her GP did not know her well and, although fully informed about the test results, had little understanding of the experience of the termination and the potential implications for her.

Linda, comparing her experience with the attention she received following the live birth of her first child, misinterpreted her GP's respect for her privacy as a judgement on the action she had taken. Her GP thought he did little because he did not have the opportunity. He was informed about the diagnosis after the termination had taken place and, when he did have the information, felt ill equipped to discuss the complexities of the diagnosis with her. He also expected Linda would ask for help if she needed it; Linda thought it should have been offered.

❏ The community midwife

Stillbirth

The women who had little contact with their community midwife antenatally were routinely visited after their discharge from hospital. Sue valued the frequent visits in the days after her baby's death and the physical and emotional care that was offered. It was the community midwife who helped her to understand how difficult the birth had been and was the first person outside her family to whom she talked about her baby. She showed the midwife the photographs and appreciated the midwife's genuine expression of sympathy.

Many women will be extremely needy and it may be difficult for the midwives to maintain appropriate boundaries to their involvement. Jane described the community midwives as sharing those weeks fully with them, helping with the physical aspects of postnatal care but mainly talking at length with her and her partner about their feelings, often staying a couple of hours so that she felt she had to tell the midwife to go home. She described the midwife's involvement as 'beyond the call of duty'. It may be difficult for the midwife to withdraw her help, especially as the timing for the woman may coincide with a reduction of other sources of support and a return to a more normal routine, bearing no relation to her needs, as Jane describes:

> That is one of the failings of the... my care was brilliant for the first three weeks and then it stopped and I think that's something I feel is OK now, but I remember at three months I felt so abandoned, so alone. And I couldn't phone anybody, I couldn't...

It is clearly difficult for the midwife to establish contact with some women, particularly if they do not know them and even more so if they are suspicious about a professional's role or motivation. Mary thought the community midwife tried to get out of visiting as she did not like mothers who did not have healthy babies and only did so because she had to. The midwife, who made four visits, described sensitively the difficulties the couple were having in confronting the fact that their baby had died and how she handled it:

> The first time that I went round they didn't really want to talk about it... She was very well in control of herself... when she was talking about herself and how she was physically... But when she started to think about the baby she was really very, very tearful and kept steering the subject away... If I mentioned the baby she talked about something else... so I didn't really press her with it and I just sort of carried on chatting, basic general things.

A colleague visited when the midwife had a day off and she described what happened on her return:

> when I went back down the next day she was much more talkative... They could talk about the baby and what had happened and the labour and everything... And they decided that they wanted to arrange the funeral themselves and they asked me how they went about that... they were just more talkative really. And talking about not just the baby but other things that were happening, family problems that they had, and problems with extra visitors and housing.

Mid-trimester miscarriage and termination

> I think the biggest factor missing in the early days was the community midwife. She said she wouldn't visit as a matter of course but I think she should two or three days after discharge. I was having physical symptoms she could have reassured me about and also she seems the obvious link to answer any concerns, especially when she is going to be involved in any future pregnancies at an early stage.   Judith

Apart from Sheila, who did not want any professional help, the women whose babies were born before 24 weeks gestation were critical of the lack of routine involvement of the community midwives. The midwives have no obligation to visit and, whilst they may understand women's needs, this was balanced against a lack of confidence in their role with women whose pregnancies ended before 24 weeks and uncertainty about the women's response to their involvement as well as pressures of work. Their apparent ambivalence about miscarriage and termination was open to negative and self-punitive interpretation by the women.

The women were approached by the midwives and told they could contact them if needed but clumsiness in making contact and what appeared to the woman to be insensitivity to the impact of mid-trimester loss meant that the women did not take up the offer. Whilst in hospital the midwife had popped in to tell Judith that visits were not routine but to ring to make an appointment if she wanted one. She was in the process of delivering her baby and the midwife did not appear to realise the inappropriate timing of her visit. When her milk came in and she needed help Judith did not feel able to contact the midwife. Similarly, Jenny described a telephone call, several days later than expected, from the midwife to say she was sorry about her miscarriage, which caused offence as she did not define the birth and death of her twins in this way. The sharp legal distinction between pre- and post-24 week loss does not reflect women's needs or the physical or emotional reality of the experience they have gone through.

❏ The health visitor

Health visitor involvement with these women was minimal. The health visitors faced problems similar to those of the community midwives: uncertainty about their role and the difficulty of establishing contact, at such a sensitive time, with a woman with whom they had no prior relationship. Jane agreed to the community midwife's suggestion that the health visitor should visit. She valued the opportunity that was provided to talk about her experience; it was agreed that she would contact the health visitor again if it would be useful but she was left confused about what the health visitor was offering and felt unable to contact her when, three months after the stillbirth, she felt really low. Jenny felt similarly confused and did not telephone her health visitor after she had left a message on her answer machine as she did not feel she needed her help.

Lisa had, with her agreement, been referred urgently to the health visitor by the hospital staff, who were concerned about her distress. Lisa was very upset by the telephone call and described the health visitor saying she was ringing because of the termination. She feared the health visitor would be unable to understand how she felt from reading her case notes and would judge her harshly. The health visitor described how difficult it was to make contact with Lisa:

I have a feeling that perhaps she wasn't ready for a phone call at that time. My feeling when I got the information, just blank information on a piece of paper, was that I had to offer something for them now, that I couldn't wait to find out, you know, in a week's time that she had fallen into some kind of psychosis so there is quite a dilemma to know when to actually phone. I think it must have been awful for her, to receive a phone call from somebody that she had never met, trying to say something about a loss that she had just experienced. And to say anything meaningful like that over the phone to somebody like that is really difficult – finding the words is difficult enough but finding the right time is another difficulty on top. But nevertheless you have to do it, you have to find a space. And to be perfectly honest you have to find courage to phone somebody to say, 'I have received something from your hospital and I am very sorry to hear that this has happened to you. We are available. If it's appropriate I can come and see you at home, if you need support or if you need to get in touch with...' and those are the things I said and she was OK at the beginning and then became totally silent and then dropped the phone in fact. And I could hear her running away and crying.

Lisa did in fact meet the health visitor again in the surgery when she gave her the photos of her baby but felt she could not trust her.

❏ The hospital support group

This hospital set up a support system for women whose babies had died, regardless of the reason or gestation. The scheme was established by the midwives and other hospital staff committed to providing effective follow-up support for these women after their discharge from hospital and includes the bereavement counsellor, who now chairs the group, the maternity social worker and the hospital chaplain. The local SANDS group had expressed concern that they met the needs of relatively few, more middle-class women and there was general awareness that the involvement of community midwives was limited. It was perceived that women were not getting the support they needed. If a woman wishes she is allocated a contact who will keep in touch with her once she leaves hospital. It would not normally be a midwife who cared for her. At the time of this study midwives undertook their work as a contact in their spare time but this has now changed. The structure of the scheme is evolving and a more formalised system of supervision has been instigated.

When considered in the context of the professional and lay support available to these women, the hospital support group appears to offer little to the women in this study over and above the expression of ongoing concern about their welfare. It was necessary to ask the women specifically about the scheme: none volunteered the information when asked about the help they had. The contact was mainly by telephone and took place in the few weeks immediately after the loss of their baby, when other sources of support were more readily available. Sue appreciated the four telephone calls her contact made. It was a way of saying to her that the stillbirth of her baby mattered and that the staff who cared for her were concerned about her but it was her community midwife and GP who offered effective help after the stillbirth. Several of the women commented that they might have made more use of the scheme had they known the midwife who became their contact.

Two of the women were more overtly critical of their contact. Judith was a private person who did not share her experiences easily. She was confused by the purpose of the meeting and was concerned that the midwife was uncomfortable in the situation:

> The midwife helped on a practical level, answering all my queries. She had said in the hospital the meeting was to discuss the maternity side and not the emotional side and a counsellor was available for that. So we discussed things on a 'logical' basis.

Judith went on to say she felt insulted that the midwife was doing this in her spare time, which she thought was an indication of the lack of importance attributed to her needs. The contact had said she would telephone again but did not do so.

Jane, whose contact also visited her at home, felt that little was achieved by the visit and described how ill at ease the midwife appeared to be outside her professional domain.

> it was about two weeks after Lucy was born, perhaps three weeks, she came round. And it was at a point where we had loads of people around. And I was becoming sort of selective about my support and she wasn't comfortable here... I felt that she didn't have the skills. And I didn't know what it was for, I wasn't very clear. I had this feeling though something to do with the practical, to do with medical matters, but there weren't any to have anything to do with... It doesn't seem to work terribly well... Again her parting shot to me was 'Contact me', but I haven't.

Although the scheme has been set up with the best of intentions and clearly may be more effective for other women it seems fraught with contradictions. The purpose of the scheme is unclear. The contact should not take the place of the community midwife and cannot provide the skilled help of a professional counsellor but neither is she a mother with a similar experience to share. A scheme like this cannot compensate for the concerns hospital professionals may justifiably have about the unpredictable quality of both the care available through the primary health care team and the support from the woman's own personal social network. A clearer definition of the purpose of the contact and monitoring of the scheme, along with the new developments in the supervision structure, may help to address these issues.

❏ Self-help groups

The professionals who cared for these women had high, sometimes unrealistic, expectations of the help available from the support groups which the women made varied use of. The literature was not always given to the women whilst in hospital. Separate support groups exist nationally and locally for miscarriage, stillbirth and termination for abnormality. The women who sought help contacted the group they considered most appropriate for them despite the differences in the definition of their experience from either the legal or the professional's perspective.

Jane initially found her meetings with the volunteer from SANDS extremely useful and described the contact as a 'a normal woman who has been through this and come out normal'. Several months later her SANDS contact cancelled a meeting at short notice. She felt let down and was more critical but her partner who was initially reluctant found the group valuable. Jane continued to attend some meetings but always left feeling that other people had a much worse time than her. She anticipated that the SANDS group might become more important in the future when other people had forgotten about her baby. Mary criticised the group for not being more proactive and found the meetings difficult because some women attended with their babies. Judith approached the local miscarriage support group several months after her termination after reading about it in the local paper. She has found it helpful to talk to women who are pregnant again and anxious and would like her husband to go.

Even if the women did not make active use of the self-help groups it seemed important to them as a source of information and support if needed. Jenny telephoned SANDS when she felt particularly low but has not pursued the contact. Linda telephoned SATFA a couple of times in the fortnight after her termination but was not quite sure why she did. Faced with the answerphone she did not pursue the contact. Lisa found the SATFA literature useful. Sue and Sheila had no contact with a support group and did not use the literature. They considered the help available through their families sufficient.

❏ Additional sources of help

Apart from Jane who, three months after the stillbirth, decided to seek counselling help because she felt stuck in accepting her baby's death, these women mainly had one-off appointments which did not appear to offer them much. Mary was referred to the bereavement counsellor as well as a community psychiatric nurse, help she did not pursue, and sought help herself from alternative therapists. Jenny was also referred to a community psychiatric nurse whom she saw on one occasion. Lisa was considering seeking counselling help. Several of the GPs commented that they were unsure where to refer the women if they needed more specialist help.

❏ Women's reactions in the six months after the stillbirth, miscarriage or termination

Table 4.8 summarises the women's reactions in the six months after the loss of their baby. All described themselves as distraught or distressed around the time of the loss, at home afterwards if not whilst in hospital. While all the women said they continued to have bad days two stand out as being particularly troubled when interviewed six months later. They found it hard to identify ways in which they had changed. Lisa continued to be distressed and depressed, unable to reconcile herself to her decision to terminate the pregnancy. She was considering her GP's suggestion of counselling help of some kind. Mary had sought help apparently unsuccessfully from a variety of sources and acknowledged she found it hard to talk about her feelings and rejected professionals who attempted to help her to do so. She continued to be tearful, describing herself as confused and knotted up, and was fearful of another pregnancy.

The other women described positively how their lives had changed over the intervening months and could identify particular low points and times when life seemed to be getting better. Due dates were particularly sensitive for those whose baby had not reached term. Returning to work marked an entry into the wider world and a return to some normality and a holiday brought the realisation that life did go on and that it was possible for them to enjoy themselves some of the time. All these women wanted to be pregnant again, feeling that being able to try for another baby was a positive step forward.

Linda and Sheila, who had reached mid-pregnancy by the time of the second interview, were clearly investing in the pregnancy and becoming attached to the baby yet simultaneously mourned, if less intensely, the loss of their previous baby. The third woman, Jane, was in the very early stages of her pregnancy and memories of her previous pregnancy had been revived. None of these women felt it appropriate to wait a longer period of time before getting pregnant. They were aware they were getting older but also thought that their feelings about the baby who had died would not change dramatically so there was little to be gained by waiting.

Table 4.8 Stillbirth, late miscarriage and termination: women's descriptions of their reactions

	At the time	In the intervening months	Six months afterwards
Mary	detached; found it hard to talk about the baby; said she was all right	no points of change; sought help from a variety of sources with little effect; at times acutely anxious about her own health	confused, knotted up, no energy; still tearful; acknowledges it is hard to talk about the baby; rejects help; unsure about another pregnancy
Sue	detached; did not realise how traumatic the labour and delivery was; found it hard to talk about it	two weeks afterwards: very distressed, helped by CMW and GP and later by consultant; three months: husband very distressed, visited grave together; four months: after a holiday started trying to get pregnant again	at peace with loss of the baby; looking forward and wanting to be pregnant; talks about the baby without being overwhelmed; continues to have upset days
Jane	numbed; cocooned from outside world; trying to take it in	shock followed by intense pain; three months after 'very low'; a holiday and a return to work; got pregnant	six weeks pregnant, pleased but not telling people; unsettled by new pregnancy, thinking back over previous pregnancy; optimistic for future
Jenny	numbed; didn't want to go out but to stay at home with memories of her babies; deep distress shared with partner	due date marked end of a distinct phase; from then on able to look forward	feels her old self; still gets distressed but less frequently
Judith	very distressed in hospital and at home afterwards	due date lowest point, very depressed and hopeless; after three months stopped talking about the baby; four and a half months: returned to work and had a holiday	subdued but getting on with life; wants to be pregnant
Linda	distressed, numbed, shocked; taking responsibility for the decision they had made	no marked turning points, gradually moving on through a series of obstacles – post mortem results and follow-up; due date; new pregnancy	23 weeks pregnant, feeling good; still sad about previous baby, needs to talk and cry
Sheila	calm in hospital; distressed afterwards at home	returned to work two and a half weeks after termination, difficult to face people; pregnant two months after termination	20 weeks pregnant and very positive; looking forward not backwards
Lisa	distraught	due date particularly difficult; continues to be seriously distressed and depressed	cannot reconcile herself with her decision, which she regrets and feels she was rushed into; anxious and depressed

CMW = community midwife

■ Conclusion

There are clear differences between the primary health care team and the hospital in the quality of care they provide for women whose pregnancies end in the second or third trimester without a live baby. The ethos of the hospital system of care, regardless of gestation or the reason for the end of the pregnancy, is that of sensitivity to the event as a major crisis and loss for the individual. There is continuity of care and women have the opportunity to establish a close relationship with the midwife caring for them. The principles which underpin the system of care appear to be:

- Acceptance of a woman's feelings and behaviour. Women are not judged for the decisions they have made or for the diverse and perhaps unusual ways in which they react in the crisis. The professional response to women is not determined by the gestation of the pregnancy or the reason for the loss.
- The reduction of suffering. Staff clearly aim to do everything they can, and more, to help.
- Individualising care. Women are fully involved and helped, in consultation with the staff caring for them, to make appropriate choices in their care.

Care in the community after discharge from hospital can meet these high standards but is generally more haphazard and dependent on the gestation of the pregnancy and the skill of the health professionals. In addition it can be hard for health professionals to establish a helping relationship if they have had no contact with the woman prior to hospital admission. There is a clear difference between the care available to women with post-24 week loss, when follow-up care from the primary health care team is routinely offered, and pre-24 week loss, when primary care follow-up is not automatic and health professionals demonstrate a lack of confidence and ambivalence in offering help.

■ Issues in good practice arising from the research

It is recognised that there are resource implications in addressing some of the issues outlined below whilst others build on changes already underway in current health care and are more dependent on changes in attitude.

❑ Staffing and training

Individualising care

Good care is individualised. The women in this study differed in many ways, particularly in their attachment to their unborn child, in the amount and nature of the contact they had with their baby and in the expression of their grief. Recognising and accepting these differences and adopting a flexible approach is the basis of good care. The implications are that:

- professionals need an understanding of the diversity of individual need
- professionals should not make assumptions about what a woman wants or feels
- health care is negotiated.

Facing the pain

Pregnancy loss in the second and third trimester is an experience full of emotion and confronts professionals with the unpredictability and tragedy of life. Helping women through these experiences means professionals must:

- accept the emotional pain of labour and delivery in the second and third trimesters
- be prepared for the reality of a dead and possibly malformed baby
- cope with the feelings that the work arouses in them
- be able to respond to women's distress
- recognise that when emotions are running high it is easy for information to be misheard.

Relationship between a woman and her caregivers

The relationship a woman has with the professionals who care for her is central to her experience. Women are very sensitive to the response of the professionals they encounter and become very attached to their caregivers. The implications of this are:

- These women valued a relationship with their caregivers, particularly their midwife, which was characterised by a more equal partnership based on mutual respect, the professional's acceptance of the unacceptable, the acknowledgement and discussion of a woman's feelings, negotiation and an understanding that the professional does not necessarily know best.
- The relationship between a woman and her midwife in sharing such a painful and intimate experience is often intense. Midwives need to

understand the dynamics of such a relationship and routinely to have access to support and professional supervision where appropriate.

- All health professionals must recognise the significance of their relationship with their patients. For example, the women valued the doctor's respect for their privacy and had little contact with hospital doctors unless there was a particular problem or there had been involvement prior to the delivery. However, they always appreciated the expression of concern by a senior doctor and commented negatively if it did not happen.
- Continuity of carer should be arranged when possible. Changes in personnel and/or location of care, for example transfer to another ward or from home to hospital, can be very disruptive.
- Establishing meaningful contact with a woman after discharge from hospital if there has been no prior involvement is a difficult and demanding task for community professionals, for which they may feel unprepared.

Seeing and handling the baby

Professionals and parents alike fear the dead baby. In this study the women and their partners differed in the amount and nature of the contact they had with their baby but were helped to do what was right for them; six months later none of the women had any regrets. For parents who are reluctant to see their baby midwives are in a powerful role to persuade or pressurise but it is important to allow parents to work out what is right for them. Assumptions cannot be made about gestation or degree of abnormality affecting parents' reactions to their baby. Professionals must be able to communicate their confidence to parents. Midwives play an important role in:

- negotiating, enabling parents to work out what they want
- providing reassurance and containing anxiety
- giving information about the baby when this is available
- supporting the parents in being with their baby.

Professionals must be well informed about disposal policy

Poorly informed staff only add to a woman's distress. All hospitals should have a clearly written information sheet on disposal policy available for staff to refer to. In such an emotive area, in which the ideas about what is acceptable have radically changed, the absence of clear guidelines means at best that inaccurate information is given and at worst that the rules are made up and opportunities for contact with the baby lost.

Terminology

Care must be taken in the application of the terms stillbirth, miscarriage and termination. The definition in law is sometimes ambiguous. In practice the use of the terms intrauterine death and induction of labour may be more sensitive and less stigmatising.

Sharing and developing midwifery expertise

All midwives are likely to encounter women with pregnancy loss of some form and must therefore have an understanding of the experience and the professional skills to respond effectively. The women at this hospital were cared for by a specific group of *de facto* experts: midwives experienced and/or with an interest in pregnancy loss who were committed to providing excellent care. The implications of this are that these midwives:

- become overburdened with painful, stressful and demanding cases; no formalised regular support is available beyond peer support
- become an elite group viewed by other midwives as exclusive and different
- the skills these midwives have are not shared with new or less experienced staff.

It is essential that mechanisms are developed to ensure that all staff have a basic level of competence and that there is the opportunity for less experienced midwives to extend and develop their skills.

Multidisciplinary review of emotionally complex cases

The consequences of providing inadequate care to women with late pregnancy loss are likely to be profound in personal terms to the woman concerned as well as time-consuming for the professionals, who are likely to be approached for subsequent help and ultimately may have to deal with complaints. In the hospital in this study any consideration of a case focuses on medical/clinical issues. The opportunity should be routinely provided for staff in a multidisciplinary meeting to reflect on a case as a whole and to consider how differences in the professional response could have improved the outcome. This is a learning process. Outside expert consultation, from an experienced psychotherapist or clinical psychologist for example, may be useful in this process and necessary in some particularly complex cases.

❏ Organisational issues

There will be local variation in the care that is provided for women whose pregnancy ends in the second or third trimester or whose baby is stillborn. In the hospital in this study women are normally admitted to the maternity unit. Attention to the following issues would improve women's experiences.

Care before admission to hospital

Diagnosis at ultrasound
Diagnosis of an abnormality or intrauterine death can occur in a variety of settings and may necessitate referral to a specialist unit. It is essential that procedures are in place to ensure that women have the opportunity for informed discussion, preferably with a knowledgeable senior doctor, at the time of the diagnosis.

Counselling at decision-making
Prior to any termination of pregnancy professional counselling should be routinely offered to women from a person independent of the decision-making process. It is essential that women are routinely provided with the opportunity to reflect on the personal implications of a termination as well as have time, when an abnormality has been detected, to digest factual information about the baby's condition.

Hospital care

Preparation for labour
All the women felt involved in discussing the management of their labour and delivery throughout their health care but said they were given inaccurate information and were shocked at the length and pain of their labour.

A range of professionals are likely to contribute to the preparation of a woman for labour: obstetricians and midwives both in the antenatal clinic and on the maternity unit. Attention must be paid to co-ordinating the professional response and ensuring that women are given accurate information about the probable length and painfulness of labour prior to induction. Professionals must accept that it is unlikely that labour in the second and third trimesters will be free of emotional and physical pain. In preparation for the delivery information about the state of the baby is likely to be helpful to both women and the professionals caring for them.

Making pregnancy loss a high priority
The women in this study were cared for by experienced midwives who were free to give one-to-one care. Women cared for by midwives less confident in their skills or who are simultaneously responsible for a woman delivering a

live baby are unlikely to receive such good-quality care. It will only be possible to maintain these high standards if priority is given to women undergoing pregnancy loss and skilled midwives are freed to care for them.

The place for labour and delivery: maternity unit or emergency ward?
Women can interpret proximity to mothers with healthy babies positively as confirmation of their role as mother or negatively in terms of the loss of their baby. The women who were cared for on the maternity unit felt psychologically wanted and well cared for. This was more important to these women than the location or the facilities. The woman who chose to be cared for on the emergency ward regretted doing so. She was well cared for within the limitations of what could be provided but staff were busy and inexperienced in labour and delivery and the handling of a dead baby.

All women undergoing induction, labour and delivery should be cared for by midwives in the maternity unit regardless of the gestation of the pregnancy or the reason for the loss. Nursing staff will be less experienced in labour and delivery and therefore less able to provide a high standard of care.

Requesting parental permission for a post mortem
The thought of a post mortem is almost always distressing for parents as well as for staff. It is usually best if parents are approached by a senior professional known to them to discuss the request. Midwives and junior doctors need accurate information about the reason for a post mortem and training in how to approach parents.

The post mortem form in use during this study included a research clause which caused offence and was inappropriately worded. The form to request a post mortem should be amended to be more sensitive to parents.

Transfer to the postnatal ward after the delivery
The women in this study were usually offered the option of transfer to the bereavement room after the delivery of their baby. Whilst this may be in their best interests and they may choose to do so, moving from the security of the delivery suite to strange surroundings with unfamiliar staff with whom there will be less contact is difficult and staff should be prepared to compensate for this.

Medical issues

Pain relief
The women had been told they need not suffer and had high expectations of the effectiveness of pain relief. There is perhaps a reluctance on the part of the professionals to accept that the delivery of a dead or dying baby cannot be free of both emotional and physical pain.

It is accepted professional practice in this unit that diamorphine is given to women in labour for a stillbirth or termination of pregnancy. The women in this study were concerned at the effect on them of the pain relief. Consideration should be given to the appropriateness of the high level of pain relief given and the consequences for the women; further research is needed.

Vaginal or caesarean delivery?

It is accepted practice that a stillborn baby should be delivered vaginally. This may not always be in the woman's best interests. This attitude needs review.

Hospital follow-up

Consultant appointment: administrative arrangements

The appointment with the consultant is a milestone for the women who, on the whole, valued the high quality of care offered. The delay in arranging the appointment for three of the women caused unnecessary distress. The appointment should be arranged as soon as possible, providing the necessary information is available, with a consultant the woman wishes to see.

Professional care after discharge from hospital

Women's needs for follow-up care (beyond the consultant appointment) will vary according to the impact of the experience, their personal circumstances and coping mechanisms as well as their expectations of and attitudes to support from outsiders. The women in this study appeared to identify one professional as a significant source of support. It is likely to be someone with whom they had contact before or during the hospital admission, who has the necessary skills and with whom they feel comfortable.

Normalising the need

In the psychologically vulnerable period after late miscarriage, termination or stillbirth it is difficult for women to ask for help. Systems must be in place for routine follow-up care. Professionals need to be proactive and take responsibility for routinely offering the help that is needed.

Planning and co-ordinating follow-up care

Follow-up care is often poorly co-ordinated. The division between hospital and primary health care and the change in personnel is unhelpful. It is hard for health professionals who have no prior relationship with the woman to offer effective care after such an emotionally intense experience. Women's needs vary and it is often hard for them to obtain help when they need it. An aftercare plan of professional support and lay support could be devised with the woman. This would not necessarily involve more professional effort – it may involve less – but the professional input could be better directed. The midwife known to the woman may be the person best placed to negotiate the package of care. She should not have to provide the help. Further research would be necessary to develop this in practice.

Pre-24 week loss
GP and community midwife follow-up should be routinely provided for women undergoing second-trimester pregnancy loss. In this study women whose babies were stillborn received a wealth of follow-up care, provided routinely. The women whose pregnancies ended before 24 weeks gestation received no follow-up care from the primary health care team as a matter of course. They were asked whether they wanted to involve the community services but often in such a way that they said no. Later they felt avoided, neglected and judged for the decision they had made or because their baby was not a 'real' baby. The difference in the provision of the service pre- and post-24 weeks gestation is actively unhelpful to women who do not divide their experience in this way.

Availability of longer-term help
A variety of sources of help are available for women in the immediate post-natal period. It is in the aftermath of the immediate crisis, when this flurry of activity has subsided, that women may need more specific help to go over events again and to consider in more depth the personal impact. The failure of professionals to deal with their own feelings of anxiety and responsibility about the reason for a stillbirth can get in the way of their ability to offer effective help.

The women in this study who had a good relationship with their GP prior to hospital admission valued the help they were offered afterwards, although the GPs expressed concern about their inexperience.

More flexible access to the community midwife in the longer term would be helpful to some women. Women must be given information about sources of counselling help. The self-help groups were of limited use to these women in contrast to the high expectations the professionals often had of the help available.

■ Suggestions for further reading

Abramsky, L. and Chapple, J. (eds) (1994) *Prenatal Diagnosis: The Human Side*, London, Chapman & Hall.

Bourne, S. and Lewis, E. (1992) *Psychological Aspects of Stillbirth and Neonatal Death: An Annotated Bibliography*, London, Tavistock Clinic.

Kohner, N. (1992) *A Dignified Ending*, London, SANDS.

Kohner, N. and Henley, A. (1995) *When a Baby Dies*, London, Pandora Press/HarperCollins.

Leon, I.G. (1992) Perinatal loss – a critique of current hospital practices, *Clinical Pediatrics*, 31(6):366–74.

Lovell, A. (1983) Some questions of identity: late miscarriage, stillbirth and perinatal loss, *Social Science and Medicine*, 17(11):755–61.

Rothman, B.K. (1988) *The Tentative Pregnancy: Prenatal Diagnosis and the Future of Motherhood*, London, Pandora Press.

Stillbirth and Neonatal Death Society Newsletter, available from SANDS (see Appendix II).

Support Around Termination for Abnormality Newsletter, available from SATFA (see Appendix II).

Chapter 5

Health professionals

■ Introduction

The previous chapters provided a detailed consideration of health care provided from both the women's and health professionals' perspectives. The purpose of this chapter is to focus on the health professionals themselves and consider their experiences of undertaking this work. Firstly, the personal impact of the work on health professionals will be considered: their views of the personal demands inherent in the work, the issues they defined as more important or more difficult and the coping mechanisms they develop. Secondly, consideration will be given to the support available to professionals: their definitions of support and their views on what was and should be provided. Although this section draws on some material already referred to it is valuable to collate all aspects and consider in some depth the health professionals' viewpoint.

Not all the health professionals commented on each of the issues identified in this section but, where they have, their views are used to illustrate the difficulties they face in carrying out their professional tasks. Similarly, not all the tasks undertaken by each professional group caring for women who have a miscarriage, termination or stillbirth are dealt with but only those on which this research has some comment to make.

As indicated earlier a wide range of health professionals were interviewed as part of this study. For the purposes of this section the professionals have been grouped according to their profession and form four main groups: midwives, nurses, hospital doctors and GPs. Reference is made where it is relevant to the status and experience of the health professional and, for nurses, their location in the hospital. Although other professionals, for example sonographers, were included in the study the numbers were so small that it has not been possible to represent their views separately here. The pertinent issues they raised have been incorporated in the relevant sections on health care.

The interviews with the health professionals focused not only on their involvement with the particular woman recruited to the study but also on their broader professional experience and views of the work. The majority of the health professionals welcomed the opportunity to talk freely about and to explore the wider issues around their work, a reflection perhaps on the lack of opportunity in the normal routine to do this.

■ Professionals' views of the impact of the work

❏ Midwives

The midwives in the maternity unit were seen by the women as providing a high standard of care at every stage of the birth and their experience and skill were much valued. Despite this high level of skill and expertise the midwives themselves talked about the difficulties involved in offering good individualised care. From discussions with the midwives the aspects of their work that appeared to be the most demanding or to present the most difficulties were:

- providing emotional support to parents
- facing the reality of pain and death
- acting as the women's advocate.

Each of these issues presents midwives with problems and dilemmas and none is straightforward. Women who are in the process of losing a baby or have just lost a baby are in a highly charged emotional state. Their responses cannot easily be predicted, nor can the responses of the midwives themselves to the pain and distress they will encounter from the women or from seeing dead or abnormal babies. Some of the tasks involve helping women make choices when it may not be easy to know either what to advise for the best or how to judge what the woman's wishes really are. Women differ in what they need from the professionals around them: some find questions about their feelings to be an unwanted intrusion, others may feel hurt because no-one has asked them how they feel. The key problem facing midwives, as all health care professionals, is how best to provide the kind of help wanted by the particular individual woman they are caring for.

Providing emotional support

The ability to develop a trusting relationship is of primary importance in good-quality care. The midwives in this sample were able to do this by their sensitive handling of an experience which, for the women, was personally intimate and emotionally distressing. The key to offering good-quality emotional support is the ability to judge what kind of help the woman needs and then to be able to offer it. For midwives this means being able to accept the legitimacy of the woman's feelings, whatever they may be and however odd they may seem, to stay with the emotions, however upsetting they may be for the midwife, and to contain their own feelings of sadness or distress so that they do not interfere with their ability to help the woman.

Coping with her own feelings

Before a midwife can feel free to give her attention to a woman's feelings she has to have come to terms adequately with her own feelings about seeing and handling dead babies and witnessing and sharing in parents' pain and distress. Taking part in the delivery of a dead baby will always be a distressing experience for the midwife. Her ability to cope with her own painful feelings is likely to be influenced partly by a number of factors personal to her, such as the number of such deliveries she has attended and her own experience of pregnancy, miscarriage and stillbirth and that of her friends and relatives, and partly by circumstantial factors to do with the individual birth, such as the degree of deformity of the baby and the degree of distress shown by the mother.

Some seemed to be able to take the sadness in their stride and not be affected by it. Two of the community midwives claimed to have little difficulty in coping with their own feelings in the face of pregnancy loss. One said she was not particularly upset by any aspect of the work nor by any particular women or circumstances; she had 'seen it all before'. Another was able to counter any feelings of sadness with her personal philosophy of looking only on the bright side. In her view losses are often for the best, a sign that the baby 'wasn't meant to be'. She believed in looking to the future, never looking back. She saw her role as being to sympathise with people a little but mainly to give the women something to look forward to. Her line was to say 'see you soon with the next one'. Whether this jolly approach was appreciated by grieving women is doubtful; the woman in this study under the care of this midwife did not feel able to approach her after one meeting with her and no further contact was made.

Others responded to the sadness but were able to cope with it by anticipating other, fortunately more numerous, happier events:

> I feel that it is all very, very sad. Very very sad emotions. But I don't have any problem dealing with those because in midwifery in four or five days time you deliver someone's baby, where there is a happy event and so it does sort of swing. You just compensate. Midwifery on the whole is a very happy time, a very positive time, maybe that's why it helps to deal with the sad days that we have.

An ability to keep an emotional distance and recognise that the pain belongs to the woman, rather than the midwife, helped others:

> Although I can feel empathy I don't feel the pain; it's empathic pain, it's not my distress. I feel that I am quite good at that. I can keep it in the right spot.

For some midwives coping with the distress was never easy. One saw this in a positive light:

You've got to do the physical delivery absolutely correctly, make sure the mother is safe from all points of view. And then also immediately turn round and give the very great emotional support, and obviously you feel very emotional as well. And I do shed a few tears quite frequently. And I think it's good because it does help me to realise that you do feel personally involved and you are not just acting like a stone wall.

Several midwives commented on the difficulties they faced in overcoming their own feelings of revulsion in handling a dead and possibly very deformed baby and how it was only with several years' experience that they were beginning to cope. For one midwife the distress was a constant source of concern and worry. She said she found the delivery of a small or abnormal baby very 'shocking' because she was not sure how either she or the parents would react. She found the extreme pain of the women hard to bear. When she had first started as a midwife some 18 months previously she said she was 'constantly in tears and used to get very down'. Although she was beginning to get more used to it she said it still took her about 'a week or two' to get over a difficult delivery.

Some experiences of loss can have marked effects on the midwives involved in the event. One who was involved in the care of a woman in this study whose baby was stillborn was so affected by it that she went on sick leave for six weeks afterwards. One of her colleagues observed that midwives 'can be affected greatly by experiences like this'.

A complicating factor for midwives is that one minute they may be sharing in the joy of assisting with a live birth and the next, in the distress of a stillbirth. The emotional demands made by switching from one extreme to the other was described by several as being very difficult:

It's horrendous looking after a lady with a live baby and even perhaps delivering a live child when you've got a lady like that [i.e. one who has just had a termination for abnormality] to look after because you've got to be joyous for that person and you've got to give them everything that they need to have a memorable confinement. And then you've to switch over into... the emotions are so far apart; it's very, very difficult.

A midwife described how on one occasion when this happened to her she had to tell the sister that she couldn't cope with both and someone else had to take over the live birth.

How to feel comfortable enough with what is inevitably a distressing experience to be free to attend to the mother's needs and not to distort them to suit the needs of the professional is an issue not just for midwives but for all health professionals.

Attending to the woman's feelings

The way in which the midwife tunes in and responds to the feelings of the woman is the crucial factor in establishing a trusting, helpful relationship. The extreme emotions that giving birth to a dead baby can give rise to and the impossibility of the woman preparing herself in advance for her likely reactions make this a task of great complexity.

The midwives on the maternity unit were valued by the women in this study for the sensitive way in which they were able to empathise with them. The midwives were able to call on their own experiences as women to help them enter into the women's experiences and to share in their distress. To the extent that they were able to do so it was likely to be at a cost to themselves as their own feelings became caught up in the women's pain. There was no attempt to hide behind a barrier of professional distance which could have offered the midwives some protection from the emotional turmoil but which may have been felt as uncaring by the women.

Coping with women in distress is no simple task. To be able to accept and respond to the wide variety of reactions to distress and grief calls for a high level of maturity and experience. Some midwives spoke of their worry about being able to cope with a woman who was overtly distressed. Situations where a woman cried a lot were described as 'terribly difficult' and 'obviously traumatic'. When women are so obviously distressed it can leave the midwife unsure how best to respond. One described her own predicament in the face of tearful women very clearly:

> I actually find people who are crying a lot sometimes... very distressing... I find it quite hard to deal with. I don't know really what I should be doing, while they are crying, whether I should just sit there and let them cry and sometimes I don't know whether it is a good thing. Like talking about babies will often make people very upset, they will cry and I don't know whether that is a good thing or a bad thing. In some cases I've been chatting away and then we've been talking about babies and then they'll start crying, really crying but I think 'Have I done the right thing in making them so upset?' Maybe I shouldn't have talked about it quite so much or perhaps I should never have introduced the subject. And then on the other hand you think maybe they do need to talk about it. You know, it's very difficult. I find that quite difficult.

Some women react in ways which seem at the time to be strange or inappropriate. One midwife found the detached reaction of one woman who laughed inappropriately very difficult to relate to. Some women appear to be in a state of shock. Midwives may have to cope with the woman's guilt as well as her distress. The unpredictability of how the woman will react can be an added difficulty as it heightens the midwife's sense of anxiety about what may happen.

What the women found helpful was the calm acceptance by the midwives of the women's feelings, whatever they were. The easier it is for the midwife to accept the woman's feelings the easier it is for the woman to cope with them; the more discomfort the midwife shows the harder it is for the woman to feel at ease. Being able to cope with the wide variety of reactions to pain and grief is a crucial skill in helping women to cope with their experience of stillbirth and pregnancy loss. One midwife commented on the problem of knowing what to say about the death of the baby; sometimes the direct approach is right, sometimes it would not be appropriate:

Some people... can't actually say, 'Isn't it terrible, your baby has died'. And I think sometimes this is called for, sometimes it's not.

Getting to know what was right for any particular woman was made easier or harder according to the emotional maturity and openness of the women. Some women were able to make their needs understood reasonably easily while others found it very hard to articulate what they needed in the way of emotional support. One midwife referred to the process of offering help as a 'constant struggle' between herself and the woman. However, this should not be viewed negatively. The fact that the midwife was prepared to enter into the struggle to discover what the woman really wanted meant that they were able to work through to a valuable shared understanding. The worse alternative would have been for the midwife to have assumed she knew best and imposed her view of the help needed on the woman.

The reference to the constant struggle is a reminder that offering effective help takes time and effort on the part of the professional, which can take its own emotional toll. As one midwife commented:

I know it does have an effect on me because although it doesn't come out very much I do remember all the ladies that have had stillbirths and I remember them all. And I remember them all really clearly. I remember all the babies that I've delivered. I can remember all the ladies I've looked after. And it's all really really clear. In fact I remember them usually much more than the normal deliveries that I've had. I mean obviously I remember those too but not in so much detail. And I think ones that I remember particularly have been particularly traumatic ones.

Another difficulty for midwives was responding to the many questions women had about why their pregnancy had gone wrong. This was sometimes not so much because the midwives did not have the answers but rather because there were no satisfactory answers to the questions asked:

Sometimes it's them asking you questions that you haven't got an answer to. You know like they so often ask why this happened and, you know, to say something like 'These things happen. I don't know why it happened. No one knows why it happened', it's almost like you are fudging really on the issue. It's not really that at all, it's just that you really honestly don't know. And honestly some people ask you again and again and again the same questions. Sometimes people also see you as a fount of knowledge as well. And they are asking you all these different sort of questions and sometimes you think this just isn't in my league, I don't know the answer to all these questions. And you sort of say, 'I don't know but I will find out for you', which is quite difficult.

The lack of feedback from women compounded the midwives' difficulty of ever knowing whether they had done the right thing. This can leave them not being sure whether the course of action they took in a difficult set of circumstances was the best one, leaving the uncertainties there for the next time a similar situation occurred.

Partners, family and friends

Midwives have to attend to the partners, family and friends of the women, for whom the experience of the delivery is also likely to be emotionally painful. Several midwives referred to the difficulty they thought men had in showing their feelings. They also recognised that the partners often tried very hard to provide support for the women but at the same time they too needed to be supported. One midwife found herself perplexed at how to cope with a man who was obviously suffering, looking 'as white as a ghost', yet whenever she asked him how he was he would just say he was all right. She wanted to help him open up but could not find how to do so.

The presence of partners can add to the complexity of the midwife's task. One described how she had to cope with a woman and her partner whose reactions to their loss were at opposite extremes:

Near the end of my training I was looking after a lady whose baby died very suddenly – she had an emergency caesarean section. Her husband was waiting outside and I had to go out with the paediatrician to tell the father the baby had actually died. His reaction was so strange because he was so matter of fact he just said, 'Oh right. Oh, OK'. And it was just so unexpected because you expect people to be weeping and wailing or at least to show some sign. I mean it was just like he totally ignored it. And then on the other hand when his wife came round from the anaesthetic, when we told her she was screaming and wailing. She was totally the opposite. I found that really hard as well. And to deal with them as a couple, with him being totally almost nonplussed and her at the other extreme who was screaming and weeping and going through the stages of bereavement you know denial and sort of 'Why me? It must be something I've done.' You know one minute she's wailing 'Oh no' and then she's wailing 'It must be something I've done.' I know the stages of bereavement and you could see her flashing through it in an instant. With her husband it was much slower and much more gradual. But I found that quite hard, she was changing so quickly.

Letting go

Because midwives are present throughout the intense emotional experience of giving birth in such difficult circumstances they develop a powerful and intimate relationship with the women. This can make it hard for them to let go afterwards, and some found themselves wanting to keep in contact after the woman had left hospital, more because of their own needs than those of the women. Those midwives without clear professional boundaries may well be tempted into inappropriate and unhelpful relationships with women.

Facing the reality of the pain and of death

Helping to control the level of physical pain during delivery

While it was the doctors' responsibility to prescribe the level of pain relief all the midwives saw it as an essential part of their role to ensure that relief was provided. In this respect they saw themselves sometimes as advocates on behalf of the women. Unlike the situation with a live birth they did not have to be concerned about the effect of the anaesthetic on the baby. However, the fact that the dosage could be increased meant that some women felt that they had been given so much that they lost all sense of what was happening to them. This was right for some women but not for others. Once again, the professional task is to judge what is right for women with different needs.

The ability of the midwives to control the level of physical pain is in sharp contrast with their ability to control the associated emotional pain, for which there can be no anaesthetic. Midwives have to help women face the reality of their loss. To do this they have to be able to accept the reality of the loss themselves. One midwife was so pleased at the way the mother had given birth that she found herself congratulating her and tried to treat it:

> as if it was all a normal birth. A normal birth and a live baby, just that the baby was asleep.

Only of course it was not asleep but dead, which the mother would know however much the midwife found it hard to accept.

Preparing the woman (and her partner) for seeing and dealing with the dead baby

An essential task for the midwives is to prepare the parents for how their baby may be when it is born and to encourage them to think about what they want to do with the baby afterwards. Midwives have to face their own fears about seeing and handling dead and abnormal babies before they can be free to prepare others to do so. Parents will have only a brief time with the baby and need to think how they wish to spend it. The accounts by the midwives in the previous chapter of how they went about doing this shows their skill in allowing the parents to come to their own conclusions once the options had been explained.

As one of the midwives said, 'there are no hard and fast rules' about what to do, which in turn means that the professional task is one of laying out the options and helping parents to choose between them. The lack of clear rules means that there must be time-consuming discussions in which parents' wishes and fears have to be talked through. The same midwife went on to say that negotiating what to do 'was really very very difficult, you know emotionally, for all of us really'.

Midwives found themselves caught between wanting to encourage parents to see the baby but at the same time wanting to protect them from unnecessary additional pain if the baby was very disfigured. One midwife described how, if there was a likelihood of the baby being disfigured, she would try to protect the parents by delaying the need to make the decision:

What I try and do is say, 'Don't make the decision now... Let me look at the baby for you and tell you what I think.' So I might take the baby out and have a look at the baby, then come back and say, 'Your baby doesn't look that bad. What do you think about looking at your baby?' ...And if they have a look and they see that everything is OK it makes them feel better perhaps. So I do work towards that goal but I'm not rigorous about it.

Midwives know that parents may regret not seeing their baby and may find themselves trying to persuade a reluctant couple that they should see their baby. Equally, they may feel that a baby is so deformed that it might be better if the parents do not see it even though they ask to. One put the dilemma very clearly:

The only thing that is really really distressing is when you have a baby that has been dead a long time and you know you have to sort of decide how to – I mean that's the difficult bit when you are saying to a woman whether or not to see her baby, whether or not you persuade her to... I would say that that is the hardest thing because they don't know whether they want to see the baby.

She recognised that, while it was usually best for parents to see their baby and to say goodbye to him or her, it was sometimes probably for the best if they did not.

Helping parents to reach the right decision can therefore require not only the skill to allow the parents to decide what they want but also the ability to provide good advice without letting the midwife's own views predominate. These difficult negotiations take place at a time when the parents are likely to feel very vulnerable and unsure about what is expected, which makes them very dependent on the advice and judgement of the midwife. She therefore has to be aware of the considerable weight her opinions and advice will carry, making it all the more difficult to allow parents to articulate what they really want to do. Midwives therefore have to be prepared to abdicate their power in favour of allowing parental choice.

In some circumstances midwives may have the additional responsibility of preparing the women for the possibility that their baby may not be dead on delivery, even though it will be expected to die very soon afterwards. The baby may still be breathing when it is born:

> We do get babies that breathe and it's very distressing. It's very distressing if nobody has warned them… It may even cry. I think it is important that they are prepared for that, and it's hard; there's no right way of telling them, but it's necessary.

This midwife thought this was particularly problematic in terminations for abnormality because of the added burden of guilt the mother could be left with. In these cases she thought it was imperative that the women should be warned that the baby may still be breathing but this was not always done:

> If the baby comes out and cries it's just the end of the world to the lady. If they are not prepared the guilt factor is huge… Some people looking after ladies can't cope with that so they don't explain it and then you have this devastating situation which I think is terrible really. That's why I think if you are no good at dealing with those problems you should have abdicated to somebody who's a bit better.

Facilitating the grieving process

Grieving for the lost baby begins before the delivery. However, the reality of giving birth to a dead baby brings home to the woman the immediacy and finality of her loss. Midwives are present from the first moments when women have to face the reality of the loss and must begin to grieve. This gives rise to another set of dilemmas: how to present the dead baby to the parents.

We have seen how one midwife found it very hard to accept that the baby was dead and we have noted that the women need others to accept the reality of the death in order to facilitate their own acceptance of it. Even when midwives do accept the death of the baby they want to present the parents with an acceptable picture of their baby so that they will have good memories of him or her. The baby is dressed and laid in a Moses basket in as attractive a way as possible. While one can sympathise with this it may appear that the midwives are denying the reality of the death, which no amount of dressing up can disguise. Women found it helpful when the professionals around them could accept the unpleasantness of the experience as it helped them to accept it too. Too much focus on presenting a beautiful baby to the parents may run counter to the women's needs to stay with the pain and to have it acknowledged by those around them.

Another aspect of preparing for the grieving process involves preparing women for the reactions they may encounter from family and friends when they return home. One midwife said that she felt that women who coped well in hospital often broke down when they left, and she made a point of warning the women that they would probably be very tearful when they got home. She recognised the difficulty that many people have in talking about miscarriage, which she referred to as 'the embarrassment factor', and tried to prepare women to deal with it:

> You know the fact that neighbours and everybody know you've lost a baby and they don't know how to deal with it. So you can say to her, 'Don't be frightened to say, "Yes, I've lost my baby but you know we are getting through it."' And the neighbours can open up a bit. I think it's very much a big taboo subject. It's awful to go home and be locked in your own grief.

Being an advocate

Midwives sometimes find themselves being an advocate for the women they care for. This has been mentioned above in respect of ensuring that women get the amount of painkillers that are right for them but the need to intercede on their behalf can arise in other situations also. One midwife described the difficulties she had getting a doctor to see the value of having someone on hand to be there for a woman who has just been told her baby is dead. She describes how the usual practice is for the midwife to be present with the doctor when the woman has her scan. If the scan shows a fetal abnormality the doctor usually tells the woman and then leaves the midwife to stay with her. However, one doctor did things differently:

> We've got one particular doctor who seems to like you not to come in and then he walked out and you have a lady who has got this devastating bombshell and her husband and nobody there with them, which I feel... and no amount of chopping away can get him to see what I'm trying to say. So you do have that problem.

The same midwife describes her role as advocate in explicit terms:

> Sometimes I'm not as tactful as I should be but I don't find it daunting to say to a consultant that what you are planning for this lady is

inappropriate. And I think the ladies have to have somebody, an advocate for them. And one of my things is I'm very hot on that and it has got me into trouble in the past. If you are a true advocate for the ladies you don't always run with the stream of things and you are going to stand out as somebody who has their say.

In order to be an effective advocate midwives need the ability to manage conflict and to handle constructively different professional responses to a situation. This raises the professional issue of the nature of teamwork and the ease with which the different health professionals can communicate and negotiate between themselves.

❏ Nurses

Nurses may be caring for women who have had miscarriages or who have had an early termination of pregnancy. Early pregnancy loss that occurs in hospital is usually a minor medical procedure conducted under anaesthetic and does not involve labour or delivery. In this study the women were cared for on busy general wards, where there are many other demands on a nurse's time.

The nursing task is to care for women pre- and postoperatively, to provide appropriate information and to prepare women for an early discharge, normally within 24 hours. In comparison to midwives nurses are therefore likely to be less intensively involved with the women they are caring for, the nature of the task is less intimate, the surgical procedure is removed from personal contact, there is a shorter period of contact between nurse and patient and the contact is more diffuse. Despite this it is clear from discussions with the nurses that caring for women undergoing pregnancy loss has a personal impact and that there are particular aspects of the work that are experienced by the nurses as more difficult or demanding.

Caring for women in distress

Sometimes I get really depressed if it's someone who is really depressed because they have lost their baby through miscarriage. It definitely affects me when I put myself in their position, how they feel.

Emergency ward nurse

It can be quite distressing sometimes, depending on how distressed the patient is and how far into the pregnancy they are and whether they have miscarried on the ward or whether it's all dealt with in theatre and whether it's happened previously.

Emergency ward nurse

Virtually all the nurses who participated in this study said women's distress was the biggest issue for them. They said that it made them sad, tearful, even distressed. A number spoke of 'taking it home' from time to time and recognised that caring for women who had lost a baby, for whatever reason and however early in the pregnancy, was bound to touch them personally. As one said, 'You can't cut off completely.'

Whilst dealing with 'routine' miscarriages and terminations generated feelings of sadness or distress the nurses recognised that there were particular circumstances or events outside the routine which could exacerbate these feelings. Even experienced nurses, who had developed ways of coping with their feelings of distress, could find themselves suddenly caught out by particularly upsetting experiences on the ward or in theatre. Some were particularly moved by the sadness of those women who desperately wanted to have a baby but who repeatedly miscarried. The nurses on the day surgery unit found it particularly difficult when a women having a termination of pregnancy was further into the pregnancy than had been anticipated, as this nurse describes:

> that is very very upsetting for everybody. I've even seen consultants getting upset about it because they are not prepared for it... The whole place will just go very quiet and it's very very upsetting... I can usually leave it behind... I was walking across the road and it suddenly hit me, and I was so tearful and upset. It was because we'd had to do a scrape the day before and I just kept seeing it and I thought 'This is awful.' I didn't say anything and then somebody else said to me, 'Over the weekend I couldn't stop thinking about that girl on Friday.' I thought it was just me but obviously it was everybody else as well. That can be upsetting. Normally you just go home and forget all about it really.

Some nurses had developed ways of coping with their feelings by recognising that nursing was a profession in which staff were bound to encounter upsetting feelings, it was all part of the job and had to be coped with. As one put it:

> It's distressing really and it obviously upsets me but so do other elements of nursing. Someone dying would upset me. And I think there are certain things within the job that are going to cause you problems.

Recognising that the job of nursing was inherently stressful was only a partial solution for some. They could see that while they might be able to cope in the short term the constant exposure to so much grief and sadness in others would inevitably take its personal toll. Several commented that nursing women through pregnancy loss had a long-term impact but added that nursing in general does and that there was the risk of emotional burnout.

Impact of nurses' own experiences

Nurses who had themselves experienced pregnancy loss could find that dealing with pregnancy loss in others brought back their own feelings of sadness and grief. A student nurse who had had a termination some months previously said that she had 'sailed through the experience at the time' only to find that some months later it suddenly hit her and she was devastated. It left her with a better insight into how the women might feel and had made her rethink her previously judgemental views on women who had terminations.

Another nurse, who had had a miscarriage, found that her own sense of loss did not diminish with time and that each new termination could reopen old wounds. Talking about terminations she said:

> A lot of people don't mind. It's all part and parcel of the work. If you see it everyday it takes the edge away doesn't it? But it doesn't for me. In fact the longer I do it the worse it gets… You've lost a baby that you desperately wanted then you come into work and you see people [having terminations].

She went on to explain that she understood why people had terminations and that she respected the women's reasons; nevertheless, she said that the older she got the harder it was for her.

Dealing with pregnancy loss on a regular basis had made those nurses who had not yet had babies wonder about their own fertility or chances of having a 'normal' pregnancy. For some this was a cause of some anxiety. Nurses could find themselves dealing with pregnancy loss without the compensating experiences of delivering healthy babies that midwives had, so the effects could be more worrying for them.

One nurse said that her religious beliefs helped her to accept the losses and made it easier for her to deal with the women's grief:

> I'm a Buddhist and I think that helps… When [the baby] dies it's only her body that dies, what is essentially her just becomes unseen and I believe that at some other time it becomes manifested again as some other life… I think every experience can be used positively… no matter how awful it is. At least you can say, 'Well I went through a terrible experience and I survived.'

Strengthened with this belief, she found dealing with women and pregnancy loss 'interesting' rather than traumatic.

Particularly difficult aspects of the work

Mixed lists

Several nurses pointed to the problem for the women of being cared for in wards where women were being treated for a wide variety of conditions and made the point that the extra distress this caused the women was an added burden also for the nurses. The nurses on the emergency ward were concerned that many of the patients on the ward, in contrast to the miscarriage patients, require a high level of nursing care. The nurses on the day surgery unit referred to the difficulty of dealing with women in for terminations in the same ward as women who cannot have children:

> On the same list we've got people that are being sterilised, we've got people who are coming in because they can't have children, we've got people who are coming in because they have just lost one... So you've got a whole range of people and it can be very, very difficult, very difficult. You can imagine if you came in because you can't get pregnant and then you find out that the girl in the next bed is getting rid of hers, it can be very, very upsetting. So we really feel that we have to, in a way, be very protective of the other people, because, you know, it's really a very difficult situation to be in... It's just traumatic – not on a large scale but from time to time you get a very false sense of security. All of a sudden it comes and hits you in the face.

Finding the right words

> a lot of the women get very upset and they cry and that's difficult to approach and very difficult to know what to say.
>
> Emergency ward nurse

Faced with women experiencing the emotional pain of pregnancy loss, for whatever reason, nurses frequently found themselves wanting to comfort them but often at a loss for the right form of words. The more upset the women were the harder it was to know what to say to them.

While the concern to say the right thing could arise whatever the cause of the pregnancy loss it was with women who had had terminations that nurses felt most uncomfortable. One experienced nurse talked of her fears that, if she talked to the women after they had had a termination, she might find that they regretted their decision. She had learned to comfort herself with the thought that if a woman cried after a termination it was an after-effect of the anaesthetic.

The fear of getting it wrong and making women even more upset than they already were after a termination was mentioned by several nurses. As a result nurses often find it easier to avoid talking to the women and avoid enabling the women to talk to them. One nurse explained how she was afraid to speculate with women how they might feel after the termination because there was no way of knowing how they would feel. This meant that she avoided saying to women that they might feel a bit depressed after the operation because she feared that this might be seen as suggesting that the woman would regret her decision. It was generally easier to avoid the whole subject of feelings and, in so doing, to deny women the opportunity to voice their own fears or sadness. One staff nurse summed it up succinctly; asked if there were any aspects of the job she found particularly difficult she replied:

> Sometimes it's just knowing what to say. And sometimes I think the easiest thing is not to say anything and just to listen to them.

Just listening to them could of course be a very positive and helpful way for nurses to respond to distressed women.

One nurse who had not herself experienced pregnancy loss thought this made it even harder for her to find the right things to say:

> You can try and put yourself in someone's shoes but you are always not quite sure of what they are feeling. So I try and be as sympathetic as possible but quite often I'm not sure what to say or whether I'm doing enough or whether I'm being supportive enough.

In contrast, a nurse who had had a miscarriage felt that it had helped her to understand what the women must be going through, although this did not necessarily make it easier for her to talk with them about their feelings:

> It sets your life back. It's the whole loss of that future. Well that's how I felt. So I see people coming in for ERPC and I just feel total despair for them. And the thing is I want to talk to them about it but then I think just because I've had one doesn't mean that they want to sit and talk about it to me... But it certainly helped me in understanding.

Choosing the right words was difficult not only because it was hard to know how to comfort women in distress or what to say to women after terminations; it could also be difficult to know how to refer to the lost fetus or baby. As one staff nurse commented:

> You have to choose your words carefully... because sometimes they don't want you to say it's a baby and they would prefer you to say it's a fetus. That's really difficult because you don't want to antagonise them in a very difficult situation.

Termination of pregnancy

Whilst some of the nurses were completely matter of fact about termination several spoke of their need to separate their personal views from their caring role. One sister described how as a student she had refused to have anything to do with termination operations but her attitude had gradually changed with more maturity and understanding whilst an experienced nurse spoke of hiding her disapproval behind the cloak of professionalism:

> You will never believe it but I actually don't approve of terminations but I would never let anybody realise that. There's a lot of us who don't approve of it either. But we just get on and do it, because in nursing there are so many things that you don't like but it's just part of the job.

Another nurse found that while she could usually cope with terminations she found herself becoming censorious when women came back repeatedly, even though felt that she ought not to:

> A termination of pregnancy for me is a very sad situation for any woman to have to come to... I do find it difficult coping with terminations when we... see a person come in for the third one; that's when I find it difficult to cope with. Because I think they are starting to be a bit blasé about it. Do they really care about what they've done? And I care that they don't care. But it's none of my business is it?

Not all the difficulties for nurses arose from their disapproval of terminations. For some the actual operation was itself a distressing experience:

> I'm not anti-termination at all... but I don't think I could actually partake in the actual act... I think I would find it just too upsetting to sort of get my head round really. I don't think I could... Especially when you have contact with the person as well. I think it would be very difficult to have that intimate contact with somebody and get really involved in that way. I don't think you could offer as good a service if you did. No... I don't think I could anyway just from a personal point of view.

One sister said she did not want to look at the remains and gave an example of how on one occasion she had become very upset when she had seen a tiny leg. When discussing the issue of disposal with the researcher she became upset. She saw no prospect of getting used to it:

> I don't want to get used to it. It's a very serious thing what we are doing. And I think the repercussions are very serious and I think... I do it in a clinical manner and that's how I cope with doing it but I don't take any pride in doing what I do.

Talking about the disposal of the remains of the products of conception was something nurses did not feel comfortable with. This was either because they were not sure what did happen to the remains, so were unsure what to tell women if they asked, or because they did not like the way in which the hospital disposed of the remains. They accepted that there was no obvious alternative when the fetus was lost at an early stage of pregnancy. The experience of the nurses in this study was that women generally did not ask what happened, in which case no information was usually offered by the nurses.

❑ Hospital doctors

The personal impact of dealing with women experiencing loss during pregnancy is in some respects similar for hospital doctors as for other health professionals. Doctors, like midwives and nurses, have to find ways of responding to women who may be experiencing all the emotional pain and grief of losing a wanted baby whilst at the same time having to cope with their own feelings that the distress of the women arouses in them.

In other respects their role as doctor places extra burdens on them and gives rise to a different set of issues, to which the doctors react with varying levels of anxiety or concern. Some aspects of the work cause particular concerns and even distress for inexperienced SHOs, while even consultants of many years standing still profess to find it hard not to be upset by some of the experiences they meet.

This section looks at the comments of the doctors in this study on the issues they mentioned as having personal consequences for them. They are:

● women in distress and their own responses to them
● terminations
● coping with the potential for disaster inherent in the specialism
● dealing with 'stroppy' parents
● fear of litigation.

Women's distress

As for the other health professionals there is no doubt that doctors dealing with pregnancy loss are affected by the intensity of the sadness and grief of the women for whom they are responsible. Consultants, registrars and SHOs alike reported finding the work personally distressing.

Miscarriage was seen as a source of sadness among doctors because it was so common and because there was nothing that could be done to stop it once it had begun. One registrar who found the distress of the women hard to bear, particularly when they cried, said he was sometimes so upset by their distress he found himself unable to speak to them. Doctors referred to different aspects as causing them particular difficulties. For some the most distressing were recurrent miscarriages to women who were longing to have a baby. Even experienced doctors were upset by this, as the following comments from two different consultants show:

What I find most difficult is dealing with women with miscarriages, with recurrent miscarriages and stillbirths. That is the most stressful part of my job, there's no doubt about it.

It's those that want the pregnancy most... The thing I get upset about is... the upsetting thing is knowing that it has upset someone else. And therefore if I anticipate that somebody is going to be particularly distressed by the news that makes it more difficult for you.

For one consultant the critical factor was the nature of his previous relationship with the women:

Women that I know personally, so women I've seen in the infertility clinic or I've got to know very well in pregnancy, when something unexplained happens, that's a tragedy. You feel personally very sorry for them and distressed for them.

The same consultant also found it particularly hard when, in his view, the standard of care was less than he would have wished:

The other group is the one where things should have been better. That makes it more difficult to cope with... you maybe have one or two a year, but it really knocks you back. The same applies if it's gynaecology; we very rarely have any problems with gynaecology, any deaths or major complications, so when it does happen it does set you back. You think, why am I doing this?

Another consultant spoke of the difficulty of being the one who had to break bad news to hopeful parents:

The sadness in life is something which is very distressing when it first crops up. So the first person who has to tell somebody some bad news, that is very distressing.

Coping with the distress

Hospital doctors had a variety of ways of coping with their own feelings in the face of all this distress. Most frequently they tried to maintain some kind of emotional distance from the women as a means of making the job manageable. The following comments from three different SHOs were typical.

I think I'm sympathetic to each individual but I don't very often take on board every woman's emotions. If you took on board every one you met you wouldn't be able to cope. I think I probably separate myself off... I'm not sure it has a huge impact emotionally because I manage to distance myself. That's how I deal with things.

You feel sympathy with the patient and you feel sad for the patient... but somehow that doesn't get confused inside you with becoming upset yourself. You can be really understanding and sympathetic and yet not feel emotional about it yourself.

I suppose I detach myself from it quite a lot really. I'm not the sort of person who takes it home with me. I just think I will try and do my bit as well as I can. But I don't really dwell on it... there's no point.

One SHO found that the difficulty of being in the presence of so much grief left him feeling unable to know what to say. Like the others, his way of coping with it was to cut himself off from his feelings:

If I have to go and see somebody who has had a stillbirth or an early pregnancy loss or a miscarriage, that's always a bit of a tricky thing. You never quite know what to say. And I don't think you probably ever get used to it. That's why I keep saying you try to blunt everything.

While experience may help to overcome some things it did not always take away the difficulty of coping with one's own feelings of sadness. One consultant spoke of the professional expectations that consultants should be able to cope with their own feelings and in doing so also spoke of how, despite his best efforts to keep his feelings under control, he was still affected by some of the personal tragedies that inevitably happen to some of the women in his care:

You feel that it's wrong to say, 'Oh I can't cope with this, it's dreadful, I want to sit and cry and it's awful.' I think there is a reluctance to actually come forward and say that because one thinks it reflects on your professional manner... so to some extent you do protect yourself and you say, 'OK, I'll keep it inside' and it does pass and it can take months; I've had a maternal death and some other things... and it took months for it to actually lift, but it does go.

He was able to console himself on bad days by remembering all the good things he had done.

Cutting oneself off from the distressing consequences of one's professional actions was how several of the doctors described their involvement with terminations. One consultant put it succinctly:

My way of coping with it is to get on and do it as quickly as I can. But I don't particularly look at... what's going down the tube and you probably find in theatre that we tend to talk about other things as we are doing it; it's a barrier between you and exactly what you are doing.

A registrar who said he had found one particular termination 'distasteful' and a real struggle for everyone was asked how he coped with his feelings about it. His response was, 'I don't know how I cope, I just block it out.' The common response of blocking off one's emotions when caring for women in distress may be a necessary response in order to get through the daily diet of other people's sorrows. It nevertheless led to some doctors reflecting on their own emotional 'hardness'. One experienced consultant recognised that over the years he had developed a thick skin and was philosophical about the nature of human tragedy:

> One gets hardened. If I was 30 and seeing somebody who had lost five babies and this was the sixth fetal loss and my wife was pregnant with our first child, I would have handled it totally differently than I do now because I'm almost at the end of it all and you have a different attitude. It's not unsupportive but these things have all happened before and they'll happen again and again and it's not the first time and it won't be the last time. We have to do our very best to make this unfortunate episode in people's lives as least miserable as possible. From a personal point of view it's not as bad as when you are young.

This resignation that tragedy was all part of life's rich pageant was one way of dealing with the pain. One registrar, however, while acknowledging that he had to suppress his feelings in order to do the job, had not yet reached the point of accepting that repeated blocking off was how it had to be. Reflecting on what the job was doing to him he said:

> I mean sometimes you worry about what you're doing to yourself... [You become] callous. Callous. Cold. Probably not as tolerant as we should be... I think you become blunted because you've seen it so many times. I think it's inevitable that you just lose a little bit of your humanitarian feelings because you've got to do that in order to live really.

However, not all the doctors were uncomfortable at the distress of the women. For one SHO dealing with the women's emotional pain was one of the main rewards he got from being a doctor:

> The only thing you can do is just sit there with them and just let them cry. And it's fine. It's not something I have a problem with. Sometimes they scream and sometimes they don't. If they want to talk, then fine, I just let them talk.

For him helping women with their emotional pain was one of the main *raisons d'être* of being an obstetrician:

> It's part of the reason why I'm doing the job... I want to develop all the technical aspects, how to do operations and stuff like that, but at the end of the day they are still people and it does matter. One of the kicks I get out of the job is when people say thank you and they say that what you have done for them made a difference and that is something really important to me.

In contrast to many of his SHO colleagues, his frustrations came when women didn't express their grief. He said he felt frustrated by women who are very closed off and would not allow him to offer them the support he was sure they needed because he could see their hurt behind the attempt at putting on a brave face.

For one consultant there was some consolation in news that to the woman would be devastating. He interpreted a 'lethal abnormality' as good news:

> To find a lethal abnormality at 12 weeks is actually good news rather than bad, very often. It's not me that's made it happen, I don't feel guilty about it and therefore there's nothing to feel bad about... we are just finding it at an early enough stage to give her all the options. So that's not so bad. What's more difficult is stuff like people with a wanted pregnancy come for a scan and the baby is dead. That is worse.

Termination of pregnancy

Hospital doctors have a central role in the termination of pregnancy; they do the operations. This made terminations a much more salient part of their experience than they were for other health professionals, however closely they too may be involved in the theatre. While there was no doubt that many of the doctors found their involvement in terminations distasteful to a greater or lesser degree, paradoxically they mostly found dealing with them easier to cope with emotionally than other kinds of pregnancy loss. This was because they could see the need for them, saw that they were preferable to an unwanted or badly malformed baby and had a commitment to offering the women who wanted and needed them the best possible service. Where miscarriages and stillbirths were seen as unfortunate personal tragedies with no redeeming features, terminations were seen as the lesser of two evils.

The procedure was generally experienced as distasteful although particular circumstances made it more difficult. One registrar described a termination where they discovered in theatre that the pregnancy was more advanced than they had expected; he said the operation was 'deeply distasteful'. He added:

Termination gets to me... There have been a couple of times when it's quite upset me... It's something that you have to do, you can't consider in great detail what you are doing at the time. At the time it's urgent and you do it. Afterwards you try not to dwell on it too much... It's a real struggle, it's difficult for everyone... everyone finds it distasteful.

One consultant spoke of his dislike of doing later terminations even though he knew the end result was the same. He added that, fortunately, it was very rare to have to do them. Earlier terminations were also seen as unpleasant. Another consultant described his feelings with more theatricality than eloquence, but the meaning was very clear:

I've done a couple of 13–14 weekers and they are – I wouldn't say distasteful was the word – I mean I wouldn't think about them later, but at the time of doing them when you see the fetal parts you think ooooh, you know, but you just get on and do it.

He went on to say that doing terminations was not particularly stressful for him because of his belief that they have to be done for the benefit of the women.

I just get on and do it... I am doing it to help the woman... Terminations are I suppose... I don't know, you maybe get blunted. Certainly I was more upset as an SHO than I am now.

He found dealing with terminations less stressful than with involuntary losses because he recognised that it was usually better to have the termination than to have an unwanted baby. He felt he could justify what he was doing, which neutralised any feelings of discomfort for him. This sense that terminations were a necessary evil was a common view. One SHO expressed the basic pragmatism of the doctors thus:

I find terminations difficult to deal with. I think it's an important part of obs and gynae... But we live in the real world and that's all part of it.

However, not all doctors were able to protect themselves from the more unpleasant aspects of terminations by accepting that they were for the benefit of the women. For one SHO dealing with the dead baby following mid-trimester termination and intrauterine death was the part of the job that she found the hardest to cope with and felt least prepared for:

Starting in obs and gynae I did find it really really awful when I was up on the labour ward and seeing 19 week abortions for congenital abnormalities or intrauterine deaths... There was a 22 weeker and I didn't want to see it but I had to because I had signed the [release for burial] form. I found it quite traumatic, horrible because I've never seen... because it was perfect. I'm glad I did because I could go and see this woman and say, 'I've seen the baby'... but I wasn't really prepared to see it, I was a bit sort of shocked that I was so shocked, a bit surprised that I was so upset by it. And then I think there was a bit of a run, we had quite a few of those; there was a couple of IUDs and a couple of congenital... and it was really awful and I was really upset by it.

Potential for disaster

An added burden for doctors over and above those carried by other health professionals was the responsibility of the medical care. Several spoke of the ever-present potential for disaster in obstetrics and at times felt weighed down by it. There was always the possibility that something might go wrong, together with the parents' expectation that it was the doctor's job to be able to predict and prevent any disaster. The worry could arise at any time, as one consultant explained:

It is nerve-racking sometimes; you see some of my patients who are pregnant and they look at me and say, 'Is it going to be all right?' I think, 'God, don't say these things to me! Don't put it on to me!' You know, there is a limit to how much you can carry. But they need that and you say, 'Of course it's going to be all right' and of course 1 in 100 is going to go wrong.

One SHO spoke graphically of the potential tragedies lying in wait on the delivery ward:

Especially in obstetrics and gynaecology there can be potential disasters with either the mother dying or the baby dying or both dying. Anything can happen; it's unpredictable but if you worked in it for a few months you would soon have to adapt because it is quite stressful.

He was clearly speaking from experience; for him disasters had already happened:

I've been put in situations in this job which have been almost completely... almost uncontrollable. Awful... disasters... tragedies, terrible things.

When the worst does happen, doctors are left to cope with it. One of the registrars in this study had had a particularly difficult delivery of a baby who had died in utero and feared that he may have decapitated it. With considerable understatement he reported his feelings of that night:

> It's scary, you swinging some dead baby's head with a sèt of forceps delivered in the night and you realise it's not going quite right.

There was also the sense that, while tragedies were part and parcel of pregnancy and childbirth, they were nevertheless somehow out of place. Pregnancy should be a time of hope and happiness, not death and grief. This, according to one of the consultants, made the personal tragedies all the more poignant:

> If someone goes in [to hospital] who is unwell and has a surgical procedure and then dies, well one can argue that it may have been expected, it might have crossed their minds, but fit and healthy mothers with so-called normal babies that go in and something happens, it's more traumatic really.

Dealing with 'stroppy' parents

One difficulty identified by the doctors was having to deal with angry parents who wanted explanations for why things had gone wrong. Parents who have lost a baby may react by being angry. Sometimes the anger may be justified if there has been some deficiency in the care of the mother and baby or some avoidable mistake on the part of a health professional. Where this happens it is usually the consultants who carry the responsibility. Moreover, they may find themselves having to explain away the actions of their junior colleagues or GPs, which can make them uncomfortable.

One consultant described a case where a woman had been told the wrong sex of her baby by a midwife; she found out at the post mortem that it had been a girl after getting a commemorative plaque made out for a boy. She was understandably very upset:

> I had to tell her, 'Look I'm afraid there's been a mistake.' And she absolutely went through the roof. And that was just horrendous. I won't forget that for a few months. And that's very unpleasant.

Often the anger will be that which comes from the grief of losing a wanted baby. In that sense the anger is irrational and not related to the quality of medical care; parents are distraught at their loss and feel the need to find someone to blame. Consultants are often the target for this free-floating anger.

One consultant said he felt very angry at having to justify the actions of the GP to a woman who had a stillbirth. In his opinion parents desperately want an explanation but often there is not one. He found it very hard to accept the anger of this particular woman. He complained that women 'want it both ways': they want to avoid medical input and be in the care of a midwife until something goes wrong and then they want to hold the consultant to account. Similarly, another consultant said it was very hard to explain to parents that sometimes things go wrong and it was not necessarily anyone's fault:

> It's very difficult to say to parents, 'Look he's a good doctor or she is a good midwife and this is bad luck, this is a bad day. People weren't thinking right, things do happen.'

Sometimes the parents' anger finds an outlet in an official complaint. One experienced consultant who professed that he could take most things in his stride nevertheless found that dealing with complaints upset him. Whilst he said that he did not in general find himself dwelling on the events of the day once he left the hospital it was a different matter with complaints. Dealing with complaints was 'horrible... I do take that back with me and I do go home very miserable indeed'.

Two of the doctors referred to the potential unfairness to themselves when parents' anger was directed at them. One consultant ruefully remarked that for the parents who suffer a tragedy it is no consolation that the same doctor has carried out many successful deliveries:

> It's awful for parents. They will never understand this concept, but you think of all the deliveries that you do, you know, your timely intervention saves babies. And that's sometimes a difficulty in dealing with parents, not only their expectation that all will go well but their expectation that doctors don't make any mistakes and if they make mistakes they are bad doctors.

A similar point was made by a registrar. He described a case where there had been a very difficult delivery and in the process the baby sustained a fracture, 'A minor injury which heals in three weeks.' As far as he was concerned he'd saved the baby's life; as far as the parents were concerned he'd injured their baby.

Faced with these apparent 'injustices' doctors may feel personally threatened and fail to deal appropriately with parents' anger.

Fear of litigation

Because the potential for disaster is ever present doctors are also concerned about the ever-growing risks of litigation. One SHO said she thought that obstetrics and gynaecology was an extremely difficult area to be working in because of the level of risk and because women were often healthy and articulate and had high expectations. If things went wrong there was further to fall.

The fear of litigation was well founded. One consultant underlined the high-risk nature of the specialism:

> I think obs and gynae is certainly the most stressful interface between doctors and patients and if you look at the medical legal side we contribute 40 per cent of all legal claims in the whole hospital. We are the largest group, so we are always getting stroppy letters or angry parents or whatever... not necessarily justifiably, because the problem in obstetrics is the expectation of taking home a healthy baby at the end and we know that's not true... several things go wrong, people assume it's because of the hospital and the doctors... 'I want to sue and I want to get some money.' That's what weighs you down on the job really.

Some doctors were concerned about the potential injustice that might be done to them if they were sued. The registrar who was involved in the very difficult delivery referred to above was worried that if the woman had sued the Trust would have wanted to settle it out of court rather than face the bad publicity of a court hearing and the doctor's reputation may be harmed unjustifiably because there would not be a full hearing with the opportunity to put the facts of the case.

❏ **GPs**

GPs are usually involved with women before and after their pregnancy loss rather than at the actual moment of the loss. They will be consulted by women who are worried about the course of the pregnancy and who may go on to miscarry or by women who want to discuss the possibility of having a termination. After the miscarriage, stillbirth or termination the GP will be there to 'pick up the pieces'. Their before and after involvement, and the fact that the women might have been patients for some time and were known to the doctor, shaped the issues that they identified as being of importance to them.
   This section looks at the points raised by the GPs in relation to:

- their perceptions of the impact on women of pregnancy loss
- the personal impact on them of dealing with pregnancy loss
- their involvement in the decisions about termination.

GPs' perceptions of the impact on women of pregnancy loss

Most of the GPs in the sample recognised that pregnancy loss could have powerful emotional consequences for women. Because of the nature of their role and potential involvement over a longer period of time GPs are likely to have a broader understanding of the consequences of pregnancy loss. Stillbirth is a relatively rare occurrence and therefore GPs' experience is limited. When it does happen it is out of the ordinary. More usual for the GP is consultation for miscarriage and termination of pregnancy.

The GPs were aware of the potential impact of a miscarriage. Several shared their personal experience in explaining their views. One referred to her patient as having been 'devastated' when the scan revealed that she had lost her baby. Another pointed to the likelihood that they will experience the loss as a bereavement but one that will be largely unacknowledged by other people. A third GP was very aware of the turmoil that the loss created in the women. She described all the many questions that the women come to her with following a miscarriage in their efforts to understand why it had happened and whether it was likely to recur. She was at pains to acknowledge that the loss 'wasn't just a little blob' but a baby and that grief was a normal response to such a loss.

For one GP the effects of miscarriage went far beyond the immediate crisis. In his view there were longer-term effects which could be masked but would reappear in the future:

> I am a firm believer that for at least some women the trauma and emotional problems of miscarriage go on through their lives and will always be a potential source of other problems, be it presented as medical, psychological, psychiatric or even social problems later on. I think there are events in people's lives that don't go away, that get brushed under the carpet and become skeletons in the wardrobe.

He therefore took the view that it was crucial to pay proper attention when it happened in order to minimise the after-effects. At the same time he pointed out the importance of the GP taking a proactive stance as otherwise the woman's distress could be all too easily overlooked:

> Obviously the better they [the skeletons in the wardrobe] get talked about at the beginning, perhaps the less impact they will have on their characters later on in life... If you don't look for it you don't find it. You can shut your mind to it if you want to.

Similarly, most GPs recognised that women who had chosen to have a termination may have a grief reaction, one probably complicated by the added burden of guilt. One described how she tried to prepare her patients for what may seem to them an unanticipated response to the pregnancy loss which they had chosen:

> Whenever I've had people who've gone for terminations I always ask them to come back and see me afterwards and I do try to go through with them beforehand the sort of emotional feelings they might be feeling and explain to them that they might feel very different after the termination and that when the body is sort of robbed of what it has

been preparing for they might be quite surprised, even if they are very sure they want the termination, how distressed they feel. And also they have the added emotion of guilt to deal with and the guilt is a very big problem. And I have lots of people that come back that I actually refer for proper counselling sessions.

This practice has a counselling service on site and the GP was very clear that women who wanted to talk about the termination afterwards needed a service that could respond quickly without the need for long waiting lists. More or less immediate counselling was a possibility for patients of this practice, underlining the importance that the GPs there placed on this kind of help.

This GP was also very aware of the variety of responses that women could have which meant doctors had to be ready for any kind of reaction. The reactions could not be anticipated from the type of loss or the stage in the pregnancy at which it occurred; it had to do with many other factors, some of which would be known to the GP and others not. The implications of this are that GPs have to assume that every loss may be deeply felt and act accordingly:

People vary tremendously in their grief. Some people have it sorted out and some don't have it sorted out and grieve for months... Some six weekers grieve as much as people who lose them at 20 weeks and it is again very variable. It depends how precious the baby is, how long they've tried... I don't think you can say that person is going to cope and that person isn't going to cope. It's very individual. And there is no way of telling and you have to assume that everyone is not going to so you want to put the same input in no matter who they are.

When women responded to their loss with clear grief reactions this could make the same sort of difficulties for GPs as the acute grief reactions caused for the health professionals in the hospital. As one GP described it:

The worst situation is when the emotions take over any remnants of rationality in these situations and you have to deal with that and particularly spilling over into general psychological problems, depression, anxiety, even suicidal feelings.

He said that when patients break down they are much more difficult to deal with and a strain on the resources of everyone, including the GP.

The GPs varied in their views of their responsibility to be proactive in the provision of follow-up care, particularly after a termination of pregnancy. Some GPs feared the suggestion of follow-up care would be perceived as intrusive so offered little. Whether he knew the woman 'well enough' determined whether one GP offered a follow-up appointment after a termination of pregnancy. Other GPs more confidently demonstrated an open-door policy regardless of the nature of the experience.

The personal impact of dealing with pregnancy loss

Manageable for most

Most of the GPs felt reasonably comfortable with dealing with pregnancy loss, especially miscarriage. They saw it as an important and often interesting part of their work and as not particularly stressful. It was something they had learned to deal with, as the following comment shows:

> I'm fairly clear in my own mind – I find it very easy, I find it very straightforward... I've seen enough sick, ill, dying babies, premature babies, stillbirths, intrauterine deaths, missed abortions, the works. I've seen them all from the hospital point of view. So I feel comfortable as well as anybody can feel comfortable with it... I've got a young family so... my wife's had miscarriages. I don't think that they are a particular thing for me personally but they may help I suppose, it's possible. Maybe they do.

Other GPs referred to this sense of having 'seen it all before' and, while few thought that dealing with miscarriages was quite as easy as the GP quoted above, the general sense that it was a manageable part of the weekly work was typical of the GPs in this study. As with the other health professionals the more upset the woman was the more difficult some of them found it to handle, but they made the point that it was the distress of the woman that was difficult to cope with, rather than the fact of the miscarriage:

> If women are particularly distressed I would find it hard to deal with but I don't find miscarriage particularly difficult.

Two of the GPs reflected on the potentially long-term nature of their relationship with their patients, which meant that they had to think beyond the immediate crisis their patient may be facing. The context of the care they offered was one of a continuing relationship in which GPs had to be prepared to live with the consequences of their responses to their patients. One GP said that when her patient had a stillbirth she thought to herself:

> this is forever – lots of pain now, the next pregnancy and child to deal with, and this will stay with them for life and they are likely to be under my care for life.

She saw it as her task to facilitate the grieving process but felt that she had neither the resources nor the training to do so. Another spoke of the unpreparedness of finding herself faced with the responsibility of the life-long care of patients:

> What you realise when you become a GP is that you have long-term relationships. In hospital you cope because you know it's time-limited; in the community you pick up the pieces for ever. Nothing prepares you for this.

Stressful for some

A few of the GPs said that pregnancy loss caused them some personal difficulties. This ranged from an acknowledgement that it was more difficult to deal with than many other problems – 'It isn't easy. It's much more difficult than dealing with a straightforward medical problem with straightforward medical answers' – through to some for whom the issue raised strong feelings of discomfort. One GP was clearly still very upset at the time of the research interview when talking about her patient who had had a stillbirth. The midwife reported the GP as being 'very, very upset' and the GP herself said that she thought it was an event that she would 'never forget'. The loss triggered memories for her of other pregnancy losses in her own family, the pain of which was still very evident in her tearful response to the interviewer. For this GP pregnancy loss was such a powerful matter that she said it had begun to cause her to question her Christian faith.

For another GP it was also stillbirths and later involuntary pregnancy losses that could upset her. She had been particularly upset when one of her patients had lost a Down's syndrome baby soon after birth and had had her second pregnancy confirmed as another Down's syndrome baby.

A third GP, also involved with a woman who had had a stillbirth, was judged by the interviewer to find it very difficult to answer any of her questions about how the case had affected her personally; she conspicuously avoided them and turned them instead into questions about clinical practice. Her patient in the study said the GP was 'awkward' with emotional issues and that she did not feel comfortable talking with her about her feelings. The reactions of the interviewer and patient suggest that this GP did not find it easy to talk about the emotional nature of pregnancy loss.

It was in discussion about stillbirth, mid-trimester miscarriage and termination that the GPs' difficulties were more apparent. Not only may they find it more emotionally demanding but GPs will have less experience of second- and third-trimester pregnancy loss. Social attitudes to pregnancy loss and professional practice have changed enormously in recent years. In discussions about a patient whose pregnancy was terminated because of a genetic abnormality a GP reflected on his experience as a medical student 30 years previously. The first birth he witnessed was of twins, one baby perfect and one with a lethal abnormality. The mother was 'protected'. She was not shown the abnormal baby, which was preserved and shown to medical students. He was unaware of the contact his patient, who was the subject of this research project, had had with her baby and said he could not predict how she would be feeling because he did not know her well enough.

Difficult patients

The issue of difficult patients was less salient for the GPs than for the hospital doctors but it was mentioned by some. One was very worried at the high expectations which some women had of the service they needed, which she thought was bound to leave them dissatisfied:

> Some people can be very difficult... And I think... there is a danger of... making people's expectations too high which won't be able to be fulfilled... I think women need a good service but I think there is the danger of making it almost too difficult to fulfil women's expectations and then I think you run into problems because you are never going to be able to do it. As long as there is a service and women manage to get in and they get the operation and they get home, I'm not sure that there's much more that you can ask for really except obviously some doctors aren't trained in talking to women and treat them a bit impersonally and don't actually deal with her.

Fear of litigation was mentioned as a major problem although only by one of the GPs:

> Being sued is now a major issue. It all hangs over you for at least 18 months and makes you feel like a bad doctor. Patients are much more likely to do it now than ever they used to be. This is reflected in their insurance premiums. Any doctor can expect to be sued at least twice in their career. This happens even if you have done everything that you could, if the outcome was not good.

GPs' involvement in the decisions about termination

There was a wide range of responses among the GPs to being involved in discussions with the women about terminations. For some it was seen as a 'privilege' to be able to help women make the decision that was right for them, for others it was a service they offered but which could make them feel uneasy if they felt it was being abused by 'irresponsible' women, while for some termination was against their beliefs and they wanted no part in it.

GPs who are comfortable with termination

> I feel privileged that I am in a position to help people in that situation. I tend to go with what the patient wants. I support the patient in whatever they want, having ascertained through counselling that they in fact know what they are about. If they are at all uncertain I will

send them away for a bit to come back to think about the problem. So it's not a problem to me.

Those who were comfortable with terminations saw themselves as being there to help the women reach their own decisions. Several mentioned the need to keep their own ideas and feelings out of the decisions as far as possible. One spoke of his aim to enable the women to come to their own conclusions and to take responsibility for themselves. For him it was important not to let his own feelings impinge on the decision, whilst recognising that this was not always easy to do:

> To a certain extent one has to try and keep one's own emotions a little bit out of it so that they don't appear. I think it's not a thing to do, to just sort of become completely emotionally blunted and treat everything the same. But at the same time it would be retrograde to let emotions get so keyed up that they interfered with somebody else's decision making. That's always difficult, getting that balance right, isn't it?

One took this to the point of never suggesting the possibility of a termination under any circumstance, but hoping that his line of questioning would enable the woman to suggest it for herself. He said he never suggested termination even if he could see that the pregnancy was a disaster. In his view women are not put through hurdles by their GPs but go through 'self-induced' ones.

Termination poses dilemmas
One GP said that, in all his years' experience, women never ask for a termination flippantly; they have always done a lot of thinking beforehand. But others, including those who generally felt comfortable with the issue of termination, said that they could find themselves losing patience with some women if they felt they were abusing the service:

> I think it can be aggravating if the person concerned appears to be rather irresponsible and uncaring about the whole thing. There are girls who come along time and time again who are pregnant again for the fourth or fifth time or whatever, in a short space of time, different boyfriend, didn't bother with the contraception and there they are back in trouble again and seem to treat it so lightly. And yet you can't get them to see that there maybe complications with this and that it really does demand that they take a lot more responsibility than they do. And I certainly feel myself getting cross about it.

Another said that while he personally felt uncomfortable with the large number of terminations he had encountered, particularly when they were among the women losing very wanted babies, he did not think that he imposed his thoughts and feelings on women and hoped to help them to make an informed decision despite his misgivings.

For another GP the whole issue of women wanting terminations was something he had never found it easy to deal with. He said he always found the discussions difficult as he often did not know the woman at all and could not give her the time he felt she needed. He was concerned at the service he was able to offer and worried about why women seldom came back to him to discuss things afterwards. He reflected on the changes he had seen in the way terminations had been dealt with over his time as a GP and was genuinely puzzled over whether he was doing the right thing by his female patients.

Termination is difficult
A third group of GPs acknowledged that they personally were not prepared to take part in terminations and would ask their patients to discuss the matter with another doctor:

> I don't really agree with termination so I don't get involved with it. It's a personal issue and I wouldn't. I'd make that quite clear to somebody. I'd ask them to see one of the partners if that is what they wanted. I wouldn't try and stop them and preach at them. But I just don't feel happy getting involved in that so I'll stay clear.

Another GP agreed with this general stance but confessed that she was still unsure in her own mind how she would react when the termination was for a baby with very severe abnormalities. She would agree to one where the abnormality was clearly incompatible with life, but had not yet decided what to do in less serious cases.

A third GP was prepared to be involved in decisions about termination but, during the research interview, it became evident that there were times when she had to struggle to keep her feelings about it under control. When asked for her views about the arrangements for disposal she became very tearful and said:

> I didn't mean to get like this – I just find termination so distressing. They just treat it like ordinary waste, don't they? I don't know how they could do it any differently. I used to work as an anaesthetist and you see it all. Recognisable tiny little hands. [Still crying.] I only started being like this when I had my own children, but that was nine years ago and it's not getting any better. I try not to let my patients see that I feel like this.

Rationally, she knew that terminations were necessary; emotionally, she found them very hard to accept.

❏ **Tensions in providing good care**

I think giving them time to talk really. And giving them as much information as they want to hear. And explaining everything that is happening to them. And just being sensitive to their own individual needs, no matter what culture or religion or social class they are. And just asking them what they want and what they expect. And still trying to give them as much choice as possible even though they might not have all the choices that a woman in normal labour might have.

Midwife

Good care is just being able to let them feel that you understand what they are going through; being able to explain what might happen, what has happened... I feel that if they feel that you understand their situation I think that's more important than anything else.   Nurse

Make sure they know what to expect or what not to expect from a physical point of view and on an emotional point of view. I think it's just to do good questioning and listening techniques, finding out exactly what they want. I mean they might not want any physical nursing whatsoever, or be interested in that... that often happens. You probably spend more of your time listening to them rather than actually physically doing anything for them.   Nurse

I don't think the fact that they are uncomfortable on the trolley or comfortable on the bed as being that important. I feel that if they feel that you understand their situation I think that's more important than anything else.   Registrar

Open-ended counselling arrangements because issues come out a lot later and it is appropriate for women to be able to return to see the counsellor they saw at the time.   GP

[Termination] Try to ensure as best you can that they've thought of all the things that may come back later and make things difficult for them afterwards. When they make their decision they're prepared for their decision and they know what they're doing and that it's been made to the best of their ability... [Miscarriage] Being available to say it's a legitimate thing to feel the way that they do and to be available to help them work through those feelings or to make some service available to them.   GP

Good care was, to a greater or lesser extent, defined by health professionals, as the quotes above illustrate, in terms of attending to women's broader emotional as well as physical needs. Regardless of the profession and the nature of the overt task in hand there was remarkable consistency in the professionals' views about the importance of the emotional aspects of the experience as well as in their understanding of the demands made upon them in meeting them. Good care on a physical level was taken for granted. Providing a high standard of emotional care was much more challenging for the staff and made demands that they were not always well prepared for or able to meet. Providing support for and communicating with emotionally distressed women, facing painful situations and coping with the dilemmas posed by the termination of pregnancy are all integral parts of caring for women undergoing pregnancy loss.

Paying proper attention to women's emotional needs during the pain and distress of pregnancy loss calls for considerable professional skill and makes heavy demands on the personal resources of those doing the caring. There is a paradox in that women's needs around pregnancy loss have a clear emotional component. Professionals identify these but appear to work within a system where the physical needs are paramount and where attending to the emotional poses difficulties for them personally because they are less confident and less equipped to respond.

■ Support

Health professionals working with pregnancy loss routinely encounter many situations that may leave them feeling personally upset. One might therefore expect them to have systems of giving each other emotional support, either routinely or at times of particular crises. However, it seems from what the health professionals in this study reported that such support was never offered in any systematic or planned way but was available at times of crisis in an informal way, more for some professionals than others. Whether it was available or not was related more to the ethos of the particular professional group or to its location within the organisation of health care, particularly within the hospital, than to whether it was likely to be needed. This meant that some health professionals who might be thought to have had the greatest need for support received the least.

❏ Hospital doctors

The personal demands made on the doctors are high. They carry the responsibility for much of the decision-making and for providing the medical care: they perform the terminations. At times they may have to carry the guilt of feeling they could have acted differently to prevent a death; they face the threat and sometimes the actuality of complaints and litigation. As we have seen in the previous section they are often upset by what they see and carry these feelings around with them, at least for a while.

Yet it is the hospital doctors who felt the least supported of all the professional groups, not that they seemed to mind very much: theirs is a profession that prides itself that 'the show must go on'. Too much concern with one's own feelings was seen to get in the way of being an effective doctor. It is hard to escape the impression that support was seen by them as a sign of weakness and incompatible with their strong, coping, professional image. Facing tragedy, death and grief comes with the job; in order to be able to function effectively doctors soon learn that they cannot afford to pay too much attention to their own feelings. In this culture they had very low expectations of support for their own emotional needs.

'It's either sink or swim'

The notion that doctors do not need support, or if they do are very unlikely to get it, begins from the moment they begin training. In the words of one SHO:

> It's either sink or swim right from medical school, all the way through and the people who can't handle it are the ones who drop out... Not that everyone can handle it, but you just learn your own defences. And in medicine there's not much support goes on really, it's quite hierarchical. It's like admitting defeat or weakness and you don't want to do that to your colleagues.

Medical man is macho man; if not he soon drops out. If he stays he learns to cover up his feelings and not to ask for help. If he has tears he is certainly not prepared to shed them in public. Medical women also learn to adapt to this Darwinian world of the survival of those with the thickest skins. The following exchange was between the research interviewer and an SHO after the SHO has been describing a particularly distressing series of incidents:

> Int.   Where do you go for support?
>
> SHO.   To the toilet. I sit there until I feel better... I don't go anywhere. What do you mean? Go where?

It is as if the idea of looking for personal support was so strange that she could not understand what the interviewer was getting at. Where else but in the toilet?

SHOs were almost all very aware that personal support was not to be expected. Only one said he thought the hospital was a very supportive environment with good communication between everyone, but he was a newcomer and unsolicitedly acknowledged that he was 'in the honeymoon period'.

'You just get on with it'

Much more common was the often expressed belief that the ethos was that 'you just get on with it'. The following remarks, all from SHOs, were typical:

> I suppose it would be quite nice to have the opportunity to talk things over. I think there is a hole in the medical profession. I think there is very little support.

> You just learn by the ropes... you are thrown in the deep end and that's been the way for the last God knows how many years.

> That's the way you are trained, that there isn't any particular support. You have to be quite independent.

> When something traumatic happens or something awful you are just meant to get on with it really.

The reference to the 'hole' in the medical profession at least suggests that some feel the lack of formal personal support as something to be regretted. Another SHO, commenting on the absence of any system of formal support, said 'it sounds unhealthy, doesn't it?'

Regretted or not, the lack of any need for support is clearly an entrenched part of the doctor's belief system and goes all the way up to the top of the hierarchy. While there is provision made for discussions of difficult clinical or medical issues there is no room for the discussion of feelings. The following comment is from a registrar:

> Yes we do discuss clinically difficult cases, why we did the caesarean section or not, but we never discuss... we never seem to discuss the management of stillbirths or tragic outcomes.

There is no room for discussion about the patient's feelings, let alone the doctor's. So alien is the concept of support that one registrar said he was reluctant to ask for help for himself because he did not want to 'burden' people and anyway 'big boys don't cry'.

Another registrar said he had known of a time when formal support had been offered to hospital staff, but he mentioned it to demonstrate just how exceptional that was:

> I suppose you get a bit of support from your colleagues but nobody gives you direct encouragement or support. I have only heard of one case where a pregnant lady died on ITU where the ITU staff were taken away after the event and given counselling and supportive treatment or whatever you call it... debriefing. And that is only one instance in seven years in acute medicine where I have heard of that kind of treatment.

The culture of self-sufficiency, instilled during training, becomes even more important when the medical student finally becomes a consultant. The need to appear above the need for any form of support is compounded by the need for the consultant to be seen to be in control, and that means in control of one's feelings as well as in control of the firm. This view could scarcely have been put more clearly than this comment by one of the consultants:

> You feel that it's wrong to say, 'Oh I can't cope with this. It's dreadful.
> I want to sit and cry and it's awful.' I think there is a reluctance to
> actually come forward and say that because one thinks it reflects on
> your professional manner. So you think, 'Oh god, he's gone to pieces,
> what's going to happen?' You know, he's not coping well and all this
> business, so to some extent you do protect yourself and you say, 'OK,
> I'll keep it inside', and it does pass and it can take months.

In the absence of any formal support systems doctors rely on the informal support that comes from talking to each other or to their partners outside the hospital. The rigid hierarchy means that, on the whole, each level of doctor talks only to other doctors at the same level. Nearly all the consultants claimed to feel unsupported, yet they also said they could talk to each other if they needed to:

> We as consultants give each other a lot of support; we sit and talk
> about things – there is no problem on a personal level between us.

They accepted that sometimes they found the demands of the job very hard to bear. One spoke of how difficult it was to cope with the feelings that come from being involved in neonatal deaths and stillbirths, yet the reluctance to contemplate setting up any kind of formal support system is evident in the following comment:

> We don't have any support group and I suppose we could... [Refers to
> neonatal deaths and stillbirths]. That's what I find most difficult
> about my job. If anything it's the thing that would make me stop
> doing it to some extent really. Because, well, that's the only thing that
> gets you down, that you take home with you, that you feel
> particularly upset about.

The one consultant who did feel supported said it helped to be able to talk things over with the other consultants as this sometimes helped to keep the sense of guilt in proportion. He found talking about the cases helpful, but at the same time he was aware that there was not enough support for doctors generally and said that this led to a lot of 'kicking the cat' type behaviour and a lot of drinking. Another consultant suggested how the support should work:

> The consultant, the registrar and the SHO have a straight line of
> duties. The SHO has to ask the registrar, so they are always talking
> every minute of the day about things, and the registrar will be talking
> to the consultant maybe four or five times a day.

This reflects the common medical view that as long the doctors are
getting help with the clinical and medical procedures they are being
supported. The SHOs saw it rather differently. For them the ethos of
showing you can cope and that you have no emotional needs meant that
they were reluctant to ask for help when they felt upset by a case. One
explained that she would only seek help for emotional matters from another
SHO because she felt it would be seen as a sign of weakness which she
would rather not show to anyone senior to her:

> It's not really team work a lot of the time. You are almost in
> competition with people sometimes which I know that you shouldn't
> be but in reality that's what it's like sometimes.

She went on to ask herself whether she thought she would approach the
registrars and decided that she probably would not. The consultants were
generally seen as approachable by the SHOs; it was nothing to do with them
personally that prevented the SHOs looking to them for support but rather
the culture of the medical profession that precluded it.

One registrar described the help he was given by a consultant when he
had had a particularly bad experience at a delivery:

> The delivery was quite horrible really and did affect me… The kind of
> support that you get from a consultant is if you do something dreadful
> they will tell you about something more dreadful that they have done,
> you know. So he would turn round and say, 'God, yeah, I had
> something a bit like that?' He told me that he decapitated a baby. But
> that helps in a strange, bizarre kind of way.

Doctors at all levels spoke of the support they got from family and
friends outside the hospital. There is a need for them to talk about the effect
the work is having on them and, in the absence of formal help within the
hospital, they look for support from whatever informal sources they have.
Whether they will get effective support from their family and friends will, of
course, depend on how good their families and friends are at giving it; the
consequences can only be imagined.

Should it be different?

The doctors at every level mostly seemed to accept it as a fact of life that
formal support was not necessary for them. They made do with either none

or that which they received informally from colleagues or family and friends. They had such low expectations of what support might be that, for example, the registrar was grateful for being told that, however bad he may be feeling, his consultant had probably felt worse. Several of them said that it would perhaps be good to have the chance to talk about their feelings but always without any expectation that it could or should be formally organised as part of their very busy work schedule.

One consultant frankly acknowledged the need for such support for the junior doctors. He said that the lack of any formal support for staff was an 'omission' and added:

> Junior doctors are with us to learn the trade and to do it. They need support when a baby is lost. If you do a forceps delivery and the baby comes out dead or something horrible like that... They need help there very definitely but we don't have anybody.

The nearest one of them came to suggesting that things might be improved was the following comment from an SHO. Asked if she thought the lack of any formal support was good enough she replied:

SHO   No, no of course not.

Int.   So what would you like to happen?

SHO   Well maybe if we were used to it it would be like what
          happens to student nurses when they've seen something
          awful – whoever is in charge of them at that time –
          you know they always get taken away and given a cup
          of tea or 'how do you feel about that?' And then they
          can talk about it. They might not say anything. And
          that's fine. But then they might feel really upset, which
          is great if somebody is there to talk to you about it.
          And to lead you.

To suggest that doctors too might benefit from being given the opportunity as a matter of course to talk about how they have been affected by a distressing experience, especially when it is practically guaranteed that they will have many such experiences in the course of their work, seems self-evident. To instigate a system where this might become a reality would mean overcoming a deeply ingrained medical culture of self-sufficiency where to show any personal feelings is a sign not of normality but of weakness.

❏ GPs

As they have also been trained into the same culture of self-sufficiency as the hospital doctors it is not surprising that GPs also share their mistrust of formal systems of support. GPs are supposed to be independent and able to cope with whatever the work throws up at them. As one of them put it:

> Lots of GPs are very independent and don't like to think they should be sharing problems.

Some were aware that this approach might cause problems for them in the long term:

> It is part of the job that you are supposed to absorb everything yourself, which probably leads to burnout.

Another said that the lack of personal support had already led to colleagues going off sick, as a result of which lessons had been learned, and the GPs in her practice now look after each other much better. Only one GP looked for a better system of formal support. He suggested using someone from outside the practice to 'off-load' on and for some kind of personal supervision but he accepted that it was 'very unlikely ever to happen'.

However, because GPs are, in contrast to hospitals, organised in practices with a staff group that is likely to remain composed of more or less the same people over time, the system of informal support seemed to be much better developed and valued. Many GPs said that they were able to use their colleagues in the practice if they needed to talk about their feelings about certain patients or events. The following comments from two GPs are typical:

> I would get support from my partners. I would actually talk a lot of these problems out when we have tea at the end of morning surgery. We always meet every morning and I would say, 'Look I'm feeling really harassed about this one or I'm feeling upset about that one.' So we discuss those things.

> We support each other as colleagues. If we have a problem with anybody or a case we will go and thrash it out with a partner. There are plenty of people to seek advice from in the practice... I have supportive partners.

One described how this system of informal support had worked very well for him when he had been very upset by a cot death. At the time he had a baby of his own at home and his colleagues had responded in a very supportive way, making sure he was coping with his feelings about it.

As with hospital doctors, several GPs said they also looked to their partners away from work as helpful sources of support.

One GP said she had no need of support for herself as she was well able to cope without it. Her competence resided in her clinical abilities and, as long as she felt confident about these, there was no need for any other support. Several said that it was comforting to be part of a wider clinical team, especially where neonatal work was concerned. They valued the opportunity to talk with consultants and others about cases and found the support they needed in that.

This GP was the exception. For most the proximity of the other GPs in the practice and the possibility of informal contact meant that there was enough support for their needs. As one GP explained they were more or less pushed into developing their own self-supporting system by the nature of the job:

> I think GPs often bottle things up and they haven't got any outlet. Very often because of the variety of cases we cannot get trained for every opportunity... so we have got to be resourceful and self-supportive and in a group practice like this its all right to go and let off steam... They would offer support practically and emotionally.

There are limitations on relying on informal support. It depends upon having a practice where colleagues are prepared to make time to recognise the importance of attending to each other's feelings and of adequate discussion. In an informal system GPs have to be prepared to ask for help from busy colleagues at times which cannot be predicted and which have usually been allocated to other routine tasks. To ask for this help is to ask colleagues to give up their time to meet one's own needs. Providing a culture can be established where this is acceptable it may work as it seems to work most of the time for the GPs in this study. It is noticeable that the only GP who suggested the possibility of a more formal, regularised system was very doubtful that it would ever happen.

But for some GPs the reliance of informality may not be sufficient. The GP who demonstrated by her tears during the research interview how stressful she still found the subject of termination had clearly not been helped to resolve what is obviously a very painful personal issue. Perhaps given the opportunity to talk on a regular, predictable basis about this and other personal dilemmas she may, so many years after the precipitating event, have made a better job of coming to terms with her feelings.

❏ Midwives

Of all the professional groups, midwives were most comfortable in talking about support and easily identified its importance. They had, as a group, addressed fairly recently many of the issues around pregnancy loss and the delivery of dead babies. They were quietly confident of the service that they offered; it was understood by all that this was difficult work and they accepted the need for staff support and expected to get it. They had a strong sense of their professional identity and had confidence in each other, in their managers and in many aspects of the hospital system, which all helped to create a supportive working environment for them.

Formal support

While the majority of support was given and received informally there was also some formal support on offer. There was a formally designated counsellor previously based in the special care baby unit whose role had been extended to include the maternity unit, to whom midwives could refer themselves if they needed. Although some midwives expressed reservations about doing so one midwife had seen the counsellor around the time of the research interviews and another had thought about seeing her but had not managed to find the time.

The managerial staff were seen to be very approachable and aware of midwives' needs to talk about the personal impact of the work on them and to be available if needed. With only one exception all the midwives commented on how well supported they felt by their managers in this respect. Two midwives said that the manager had set up a debriefing meeting promptly after distressing incidents and gave this as an example of the caring environment in which they worked. They felt that they could always ask for such a meeting if they needed to. The following was typical of the midwives' views of their managers:

> I'd go and talk to [my manager] about it. She is lovely; she is very, very approachable... She is always there and she will always make time for you to go and talk about things. It may not be on the day that you want to talk to her but she is always there and I feel that... I've never had any problems. I know that if I'd any problems I could go to her and say 'Can I have a chat?' And I know she will make time if she can. That's really good.

Several referred to how useful it was that the hospital employed a bereavement officer. While she was not herself used as a support by the midwives in the same way as they used their colleagues or managers they said that it was a source of support to them that they had someone who would take over all the arrangements for disposal and funerals, and so on, which would otherwise have fallen to them.

The formal support that was available had to be triggered by the midwives, that is, it was available on demand rather than as part of the normal working routine. Several said that they preferred this to an arrangement of regular formal group meetings, which they said had been tried unsuccessfully in the past.

Informal support: 'cuddles in the sluice'

While they were appreciative of the formal support that was available the midwives did not seem to want this to be put on a more organised footing, largely because they were very satisfied with their own system of informal support. Although the manager was identified as being supportive, the main support network lay almost entirely between the midwives themselves.

On the delivery ward they were unanimous in their belief that their informal support arrangements were good. People knew what you were doing and acknowledged that it was difficult, offering support without being prompted. Being asked how you were and offers of practical help were highly valued. There was an understanding that midwives could have assistance in what were technically straightforward deliveries if they felt they wanted the moral support and if staffing allowed. It was accepted that it was reasonable to ask for help with aspects of the care that were not straightforward. Midwives expected, where possible, to care for only one woman at a time if she was losing her baby. Of the many examples the following two catch the flavour of the way the midwives felt cared for and supported by their colleagues:

> They are all very very good at looking after the midwife who is looking after a lady like that. When it's quiet they will make sure that you will get a break, they will make sure that you get a cup of tea and they look after you. They more frequently ask you, 'How are you? Is there anything that you want to talk about?' And at the end of a situation there is always somebody there to give you a hug. So I think it's really quite good there. I think you get a lot of peer group support. I've got no complaints at all.

> We actually have a very good system... whereby any midwife who is caring for somebody who has had a sad circumstance... we have a very good relationship between all the midwives whereby everybody is really supportive and keeps on saying, 'Are you all right? Is there anything I can do for you?'... It's very very good. We can meet with our colleagues and sort of help ourselves through it as well.

Doctors too were sometimes helpful when on duty with the midwife by talking about difficult deliveries although this could not be relied on. When it happened it was often much appreciated:

> I found the consultant very, very supportive. He was absolutely brilliant. He was really brilliant and he was very supportive of me.

On the postnatal ward, where midwives came into contact with parents in the bereavement room, staffing levels were much reduced, which led to rather less satisfaction with the support available. There was little time available to debrief and not much choice of who to do it with, one midwife having a sense that much of what was offered was 'cursory'.

Support meant several different things to midwives. It was shown in the awareness of the managers, who not only made themselves available if needed but also took the initiative in calling special meetings after tragic events, but above all it meant having colleagues who were open to their needs and offered help and comfort at difficult times or, as one of them put it, 'cuddles in the sluice'.

Less often mentioned was the opportunity to talk about how their work affected them personally. A community midwife said that she had found it a 'tremendous help' to talk something through with a colleague and that this was very necessary given the nature of the work but this was not how support was usually seen. When it was mentioned as an important part of what support could be it was also said that it was difficult to arrange for any length of time because everyone was usually so busy on the wards and shifts broke up the continuity of colleague groups. Gestures of concern, offers of help and hugs take up little time and can all be given no matter how busy people are; they were much valued. They are not, however, the same as having the opportunity to talk through the impact of being involved in a highly charged emotional incident of pregnancy loss or the longer-term effects of being involved in many such incidents. Perhaps this lay behind the comment from the midwife who said that she felt much of the support was 'cursory'.

Family and friends

Away from the ward midwives felt a reluctance to discuss some of what they had seen. 'It sounds like something out of a horror film' was one comment and those family and friends who took an interest in their work could not be expected to understand it. One said she talked things over in depth with her mother but the more frequent comment was on the limitations of using friends and family for support. One found it difficult to explain what the work was really like; another who had tried to tell her partner about a distressing experience found the response 'these things happen, why are you getting upset?' less than helpful. Another midwife said that she lived on her own so was dependent on the support she got from colleagues.

Some people may be very fortunate in the support and help they get from their family and friends but, as these examples show, some may not and it is far too chancy a system to be relied upon to do the work of providing effective support.

Organisational factors facilitating support

It is perhaps not surprising that midwives have addressed their needs for support. They have a stressful role to play but also have organisational advantages over other groups by being located for the most part in one ward and, like GPs, have a group of colleagues whose personnel remain reasonably constant over time. As one explained, the improvements in the provision of support had come about had because they had been able to make their demands known.

It was noticeable that the community midwives felt less well supported than those in the hospital, largely because they did not have the benefit of a group of colleagues around them at critical times. One who described a very good experience of being supported through a stillbirth was referring to her experience in the hospital rather than as a community midwife. One community midwife said she did not need any support, the only one of all the midwives to say so; perhaps she had had to learn to do without it. Another said that her colleague had had to go off sick for a while after a distressing experience, which she attributed to the lack of support available to her. The relative isolation of community midwives seems to be a key factor in the difference between them and their hospital colleagues in how well supported they felt.

❏ Nurses

As with the midwives, the extent to which nurses felt supported was partly a function of where in the hospital they worked. Those who worked in the three main wards where pregnancy loss occurred generally felt themselves to be very well supported by both the ward sister and their immediate colleagues. There were three nurses who worked more independently in the recovery room, EPAC and outpatients department. One felt very isolated, undervalued and unsupported. Of the two others their experience of support depended very much on their relationship with the doctors. One felt very supported by her doctors; the other felt as though she was the one who was providing support to the parade of junior doctors who passed through her unit.

Formal support

One of the wards had regular monthly meetings for the nurses, at which they felt it was possible to discuss 'anything and everything'. This included talking about the effects of distressing cases and was seen as a valuable source of support. It was also possible for meetings to be called on an *ad hoc* basis if necessary, for the same purpose. Nurses also felt that the ward sister was always available and more than willing to talk things over with any nurse who might be experiencing difficulties with the work. Not surprisingly, this ward was seen by the nurses as being very supportive. However, the ward sister did not feel that she had much support for herself other than from other sisters; there was no formal system that she could call on.

The other two wards did not have regular meetings. In one, support was also offered on demand by the ward sister and was greatly valued. In the other nurses were aware that they could have access to the hospital's counsellors and the ward had a procedure for calling debriefing meetings if 'something really awful happens'. However, neither of these formal facilities was often used.

Informal support

On all three wards the usual way in which nurses were helped to get through the 'really awful' events that sometimes occurred was by the informal support of the other nurses and the ward sisters. Most nurses thought the level of support they could rely on was at least adequate and sometimes very good:

> We're very close colleagues so perhaps that's why we don't feel that stressed because we can talk to each other about anything. So we are very close. I think it's a very close unit actually. It's one of the closest I've worked on. If we are upset or anything has... you know there is somebody you can go and talk to or you feel at ease having a good cry about it in the toilet and [the ward sister] is a very sympathetic and compassionate person anyway. Or you can easily just come into her and she will just sit you down and just talk to you and that's great. So you've always got that support. It's superb. Not just from [sister] but from the others.

The nurses felt that they were able to acknowledge their limitations and admit to difficulties without this being seen as a sign of weakness. In stark contrast to the ethos of infallibility cultivated by the doctors, nurses appreciated the freedom they were given by their ward sisters to express their doubts and concerns and to have them listened to without it being held against them. One nurse described how this acceptance of their vulnerability was valued so much by them that in effect it worked as a spur to them to give of their best in return:

> Sister is very good and offers a lot of support for everybody and in response everybody gives her support back by which I mean carrying out the work to their best ability. And I think at the end of the day that's probably the most important thing. I mean at least we work in an environment where we are not afraid to say, 'I can't do this' and you are not thought any less of, which is quite important.

While valuing the considerable support that fellow nurses were able to give there was also an awareness of the limitations of relying on this kind of informal support when time was at a premium and everyone was usually seen as being very busy. Sometimes it was just not possible to take time out to reflect on one's own feelings as the list had to be got through and patients' demands met. If one's immediate colleagues were under pressure nurses did not want to add to it by burdening them still further with their own worries. The following was said by a student nurse but the recognition that lack of time meant that support might not be forthcoming was echoed by others more experienced:

> Sometimes you don't always have time to sit down and reflect on things with your preceptor because they have got their own things and it is a busy ward so you haven't got a half an hour to sit down and say, 'I was really upset today.' And quite often you take it home with you. And I've got a friend, who is a fellow student and we actually talk quite a lot about what has gone on during the day, whatever it maybe. And get a lot of our stresses off before we go home.

The lack of time to deal with one's feelings at the time, due to the pressure of work, meant that nurses sometimes found that they had a delayed reaction. One described that she had found herself unaccountably crying the next day on the way home from work, which had puzzled her until she saw it as a response to the stress of the previous day.

One dissenting voice acknowledged that there was informal support but thought it was inadequate. She thought there was a culture now being encouraged by the higher management that it was no longer acceptable to be off sick. There has been much sick leave among nurses, which she saw as one way in which nurses reacted to the stress of the job, but now there is pressure not to be off sick or it becomes a disciplinary offence. She thought that nurses should be able to have 'mental health days' that they could take when things were getting too much.

For most nurses the informal support from colleagues worked well despite the limitations. They mostly said that they preferred it to the idea of having people brought in from outside or of having special support groups, which some said had been tried before but without much success. They thought the best kind of support was from people they knew and trusted. One ward also saw themselves as 'a pretty tough lot' who could cope with their own problems. What some said they would value was more opportunity just to talk over the events of the day. Once again, time was seen as the inevitable enemy.

Family and friends

For most nurses support outside work was important and came most usefully from friends who were themselves in the profession and preferably on the same hierarchical level. This was because the work could not easily be discussed with some people because it may be too gruesome, there were issues of confidentiality and it needed to be understood in the context of the rest of the work. Two said they could talk to members of their family even though they were not in the profession and they considered themselves fortunate in being able to do so.

■ Conclusion

With the exception of the hospital midwives and some of the nurses the formal support available to health professionals in the health care system is inadequate. Health professionals by and large work within a macho culture where they are expected to maintain their objectivity and not be distressed. Whilst informal support has its place and working in an open environment where problems are shared was perceived as helpful it is all too easy for problems to be passed around and issues to remain unresolved. A lot of support comes from family and friends, which raises issues of confidentiality. This study did not look at the experience of staff families; the emotional costs on family life can only be speculated upon.

There is no formalised opportunity for health professionals to reflect on either the content of their work or on the personal consequences of doing it. Reflection on a health professional's own coping mechanisms in the face of distressing events and consideration of personal strategies to mitigate or limit aspects of their coping style which are unhelpful to patients does not occur.

Staff will be unable to meet women's needs if the system they work in denies their own needs for support and care. High-quality health care is multidisciplinary and will include:

- automatic debriefing after particularly distressing events
- a review process in which alternative courses of action in individual cases can be considered
- a mechanism for acknowledging the personal impact of the everyday grinding, repetitive distress and disappointment with which many staff have to deal
- a mechanism for enabling staff to reflect on their own coping mechanisms and develop alternative strategies if appropriate.

A well-managed system that addresses these issues will have lower levels of staff sickness, complaints and litigation and will more easily maintain both the service and the clinician's values, enabling staff to keep on caring.

■ Suggestions for further reading

Bond, M. (1995) *Stress and Self Awareness: A Guide for Nurses*, Oxford, Butterworth Heineman.

Butterworth, C. A. and Faugier, J. (1992) *Clinical Supervision and Mentorship in Nursing*, London, Chapman & Hall.

Hawkins, P. and Shoet, R. (1989) *Supervision in the Helping Professions*, Milton Keynes, Open University Press.

Kohner, N. (1994) *Clinical Supervision in Practice*, London, King's Fund.

NASS (1992) *A Charter for Staff Support for Staff in the Health Care Services*. Available from National Association for Staff Support, 9 Carandon Close, Woking, Surrey, GU21 3DU. Tel: (01483) 771599.

Schoett, J. (1996) The needs of midwives: managing stress and change, in Kroll, D. (ed.), *Midwifery Care for the Future: Meeting the Challenge*, Eastbourne, Baillière Tindall.

Chapter 6

The dilemmas in individualising care

■ **Personal, professional and organisational definitions of experience**

❏ **The diversity of women's experience**

The experiences of the women in this study amply illustrate that the loss of a pregnancy, whatever the gestation or the reason for it, is unique for each individual. Women bring their own history and personality with them. They differ in their expectations, in the meaning the pregnancy has for them, in their reactions at the time as well as over time and in the specific details of the health care that is appropriate for them.

Miscarriage may be experienced by women as a loss or purely in terms of crisis and trauma. Laura was relieved she miscarried and was ultimately grateful she did not have to follow through her decision to terminate her pregnancy whilst Ann was traumatised. She grieved the loss of her baby, her identity as a parent was impaired and her hopes for the future were dashed.

Early termination is normally experienced as a relatively short-term crisis but a few women will define their experience in terms of loss. For Ros the early termination of an unwanted pregnancy was a relief, a medical solution to an 'illness', clarified her feelings about a second child and, although fleetingly reflected on, was soon in the past. Debbie however experienced the termination as the loss of her baby and agonised over the decision, her potential as a parent and the impact on her relationship with her partner. In addition her pregnancy revived unresolved problems from her past.

In contrast the women whose pregnancies ended in the second or third trimesters all defined their experience, to a greater or lesser extent, in terms of loss. It is the fact of labour and delivery that differentiates early and late pregnancy loss. It is possible to experience miscarriage and early termination as an illness or as a medical event and little, or even nothing, to do with pregnancy or a baby. Regardless of the attachment she has formed prenatally with the baby it is very difficult for a woman to go through labour and delivery and maintain that position.

Although stillbirth, late miscarriage and termination were always experienced as a loss the women varied in their attachment to their unborn child and the extent to which and the ways they mourned their baby. They particularly differed in the amount and nature of the contact they had with their baby, how public or private they were in the expression of their grief and their readiness for another pregnancy. Sheila was straightforward and matter-of-fact about her baby's abnormality – 'this one was not meant to be' – and anxious to continue with another pregnancy whilst Linda, who also soon embarked on another pregnancy, simultaneously and actively mourned the baby she had lost. Jane maximised the contact she had with her stillborn baby and organised a well-attended funeral. Mary, in contrast, had little contact with her baby and expressed her grief privately whilst Sue wanted to put the stillbirth of her first baby behind her and defined the experience as 'a step on the road to a healthy baby'.

❏ Organisational definitions

A comparison of the organisational definition with women's experiences provides a framework within which the strengths and weaknesses of care from the viewpoint of the individual woman can be understood. The organisational definitions of miscarriage, early termination and later losses, as reflected in the system of health care that is provided, are more rigid than the women's or the professionals' definitions.

Miscarriage is viewed in organisational terms as a minor medical emergency, a one-off event with no context, and health care is compartmentalised and fragmented. Similarly, early termination is viewed as a minor medical event but health care is additionally characterised by respect for women's privacy and acceptance of the decision she has made. The study amply illustrates how these definitions suit some women but not others.

In contrast health care for late miscarriage, termination and stillbirth is characterised by sensitivity to the individual nature of the event as a major crisis and loss and by acceptance and understanding. With this ethos of care it is predictable that the women in this study in the second and third trimesters of pregnancy were more likely to feel well cared for than those who had had an early miscarriage or termination of pregnancy.

Women are more likely to feel positive about their health care if the organisational definition of the experience, as reflected in the way care is organised, fits with their own definition of the experience. It is clear that, in this study, there is a greater fit between the personal and organisational definitions for women whose pregnancies ended in the second and third trimesters and a greater dissonance for those whose pregnancies ended in the first. However sensitive, competent and experienced professionals are, if they work within a system that denies the reality of a woman's experience, it will be much more difficult for them to meet a woman's needs effectively, which may also be at considerable cost to themselves.

❑ Flexibility: the professionals' perspectives

Contrary to my assumptions when I started this research there is no evidence from the health professionals who contributed to this study of a wide divergence in understanding between women and health professionals of the experiences of individual women or of miscarriage, stillbirth or termination in general. The original hypothesis that health professionals operate a rather crude model of understanding based on the gestation of the pregnancy or whether the pregnancy ended voluntarily or not is wrong. There is ample evidence that health professionals in general operate a much more flexible and sophisticated model in tune with the women's own experiences based on their personal and professional experience of pregnancy. Many staff gave examples of a friend's experiences of miscarriage or referred to their own experience of pregnancy or parenthood when discussing their ideas about pregnancy loss or making sense of their patient's experience as well as sharing their professional experience of caring for women in similar circumstances.

This does not mean that professionals always get it right. There are many examples throughout this study of women feeling misunderstood by health professionals or of failing to get the help they need. However, the reason for the misunderstanding is not that health professionals have a poor, misinformed or inaccurate grasp of the nature of miscarriage, termination or stillbirth for women in general but for other reasons. Health professionals may fail to communicate effectively their understanding to women either because they lack the confidence and the skills and or because they work in a system which does not allow or makes it very hard for them to do so. It is clear, for example, that the nursing staff on the day surgery unit and the emergency ward had an excellent grasp of the experience of early termination of pregnancy and miscarriage respectively but many of them eloquently described the inadequacy they felt in talking to women about it. Whilst the women may have felt well cared for they said, 'it was all so unspoken' or felt ignored.

Health professionals may underestimate their own skill and the opportunity they have to provide a women with the help she needs. For example, the nurse in the recovery area was the only person who engaged with Val and who recognised how she was feeling but, because it was not her job, she did not reach out to her and an opportunity was missed. Val had no idea how accurately this nurse understood what she was going through. There are also examples of unintended insensitivity, for example the consultant who allegedly commented on savings to the NHS when he discussed with Linda the abnormality of her baby prior to making the decision to terminate the pregnancy.

Throughout the study there are many examples of health professionals making incorrect assumptions about what an individual is feeling or wants and therefore, from a woman's point of view, of getting it wrong. This is more likely to occur in highly charged situations when attempts are made to avoid disturbing events, for example the consultant who thought Sheila would be shocked by her very deformed baby and would be unable to spend much time with the baby, or the staff who thought, when a scan confirmed her miscarriage, that Pauline was on her own because she wanted to be.

These are examples of a professional's own feelings getting in the way of understanding an individual's viewpoint often when the situation is distressing and the professional is working in a very pressured system with little time to give, of taking things at face value and of making general assumptions about how other people will react without checking out with the woman whether the professional has got it right. These examples are not indicative of a wide gap in understanding between professional and patient.

■ The basis for good care

When women's experience is so diverse applying a set formula or package of care is clearly likely to be unhelpful for many women; they need care that is appropriate for them. Whilst guidelines may be helpful in reminding health professionals of things that have to be done, often when time is limited and feelings are running high, if they are rigidly adhered to and become relied upon as set lists of what to do, they become counter-productive and inhibit the individualising of care. Guidelines for good care can become a modern tyranny akin to the old-fashioned view that the professional knows best. It was the process of care of involvement and participation and of greater equality with their caregiver, rather than the specifics of the care, that was important for these women. They felt well cared for when:

- health care was individualised
- care was negotiated and not imposed upon them
- professionals engaged with them
- the emotional aspects of pregnancy loss were acknowledged and not avoided.

❏ The individual

Respecting and understanding the individual nature of experiences are fundamental. The professional does not necessarily have to know what a particular woman is feeling or how she is interpreting the experience but does have to communicate that individuals experience these things differently; she has to be accepting rather than prescriptive. Women undergoing pregnancy loss need to feel understood and accepted for themselves and not to have reactions imposed upon them.

❑ Negotiation

Negotiating care is about providing women with sufficient information so that they can be involved in making decisions about their care. It involves consultation, explanation, giving choice as well as a change in the power balance in the relationship between patient and professional. Professionals do not necessarily know what is best. However, it does not mean that professionals abdicate their responsibility, embrace the consumer culture and give women complete choice. Professionals have knowledge, skills and expertise and a responsibility to ensure the well-being of their patient.

A realistic understanding of the limitations of choice is essential. In many instances there are few choices available. It is inappropriate to give women a choice when one of the options will automatically result in a lower standard of care. For example, it was predictable that difficulties would arise when Lisa was allowed to choose to be cared for by less experienced staff on the emergency wa.d. She did not know what she was choosing and was too distressed to be making decisions. In addition there will always be some women who want professionals to make decisions on their behalf.

Women often feel helpless when a miscarriage or fetal death is diagnosed and those who have opted for a termination of pregnancy may feel circumstances dictate that they have no real choice. Involving women in making decisions about their care may help them to regain a sense of control and so have psychological benefits beyond the immediate decisions that are made.

❑ The relationship between a woman and her carers

Individualised care can only occur within the context of a positive and helpful relationship between patient and professional. However brief the contact it is the quality of the relationship between the woman and the health professional that is significant, the fact that health professionals present themselves as human beings, give of themselves, are open to their own and the woman's feelings and enter her world. Caregivers who listen, understand and respond empathically help the most. In this sense good care is an interactive process.

The midwives assisting the women during labour and delivery were clearly able to provide this relationship. They were involved with the woman over a longer period of time, often for more than one shift. Even when contact is short and task-specific the nature of the relationship between patient and professional is important. Jane valued the contact with the anaesthetist who administered the epidural when she was in labour. Katy appreciated the way the sonographer told her she was miscarrying again. For the women who miscarried in early pregnancy it was the absence of this relationship and the lack of feeling they were understood that it engenders that made them feel so negative about their care.

❑ The emotional nature of the experience

Miscarriage, stillbirth and the termination of pregnancy are experiences that are full of emotion and may arouse powerful feelings for both woman and staff. Pregnancy loss arouses fears about the fragility and unpredictability of life which, in our normal day-to-day existence, we naturally try to avoid. It confronts us with what can be considered unacceptable, for example the tragedy of miscarriage and stillbirth, the complexity and responsibility of decision-making for the termination of pregnancy, the distastefulness of many procedures and the perceived ugliness of a malformed preterm baby. Facing and not denying or avoiding the emotional reality whilst containing the fears and anxieties that are aroused is the basis of good care.

It is natural and only human to want to avoid painful situations or to want to make it better in some way. Sometimes it just seems too sad. For example, the midwife who assisted at the birth of Jane's baby found it hard to accept that such an apparently healthy and perfect baby was dead and described the baby as asleep. Another midwife who could not face the brutality of death told the mother her baby would be like he was asleep. The mother was then shocked by the state of the baby.

At other times it is just too distasteful or shocking. The widespread ignorance about the remains of the pregnancy after early miscarriage and disposal procedures can be interpreted in general as a means of protecting staff from having to know about and explain to women something that is in reality extremely distasteful. The fact that some staff are prepared to tell white lies and make up what happens in order to make procedures more acceptable confirms this. The registrar who said he explained miscarriage to women by playing down the reality of the fetus, or the professional who failed to prepare women adequately for second- or third-trimester delivery, is unlikely to be helpful to women. Pretending something is different from how it is, when the truth is revealed, results in women feeling let down and conned.

Care can be organised in such a way that the emotional reality is acknowledged and so is facilitative to both women and staff or in a way that denies the emotional nature of the experience. For example, for the early termination of pregnancy, the ethos of respect for the difficult decision that is made means that the emotional nature of the experience is ignored. Open discussion about the decision, the procedures and the woman's feelings about it are largely avoided by the way in which health care is organised and the attitudes of those who provide it.

Similarly, the disjointed care for women who miscarry early in pregnancy means that the emotional nature of the experience is rarely addressed. When care is compartmentalised in this way it is easy for staff to 'pass the buck' to avoid undertaking an aspect of the work they find more difficult, justifying this by assuming that someone else in the chain of care will do it. The SHOs assumed that the nurses talked in more depth to the women who miscarried. The nurses excused themselves from this task on the grounds that the health visitors were informed, the women could go to their GPs and the support groups were very good.

In contrast the continuity and one-to-one midwifery care provided for those delivering a baby in the second and third trimesters enabled a safe relationship to be developed with the midwife in which the sadness of the situation could be faced.

There are many examples of when health professionals' own reactions get in the way of the care they are able to provide. The GP who was unable to discuss the issues around the early termination of pregnancy with the interviewer without becoming tearful had failed to handle appropriately the woman's initial request for a termination of pregnancy. The GP was distressed by her experience some years earlier as an anaesthetist at an abortion clinic. The midwife, who was so upset at the diagnosis of the stillbirth of Jane's baby, was clearly prevented, by her own distress and desire to find the baby's heartbeat, from responding empathically and competently to Jane.

There are also many instances where health professionals, fearful of how women might respond, are ill at ease with the expression of emotions and unsure of what to say or do. The nurses on the emergency ward and the day surgery unit frequently said they 'feared to probe'. They kept communication with women at a superficial level because they feared they would make things worse for women by reminding them of difficulties that were best kept under the surface and they feared they would not know what to do if the woman got upset.

There are few examples in this study of the overt denial of the emotional reality of the experience that, until relatively recently, were frequent sources of women's complaints. Judith's community midwife took the 'don't wallow in it, it's just for the best, look on the bright side, it wasn't meant to be, I'll see you with the next one' approach. Needless to say Judith did not appreciate this complete denial of the emotional reality of her grief for the loss of her baby at 23 weeks gestation, her third miscarriage, but her experience was rare.

Individual health professionals can understand their own reactions and respond on an emotional level to women or they can avoid the feelings altogether. A failure to face the emotional nature of the experience, to contain and make safe the strong feelings that are engendered, results in women feeling uncared for and making complaints, ultimately leading to litigation, a fear that increasingly underpins much of obstetric practice.

■ Overcoming the obstacles in providing good care

❏ Organisational issues

The organisation can limit or facilitate the quality of care that is helpful to women. There are clearly organisational constraints on improving the service. Without an increase in funding to provide more staff or to improve facilities little can be done. If women are admitted to the maternity unit when the ward is busy and no more staff are available the one-to-one care provided for the women in this study will be impossible. Providing an independent counselling service for women requesting the termination of a pregnancy or for those considering a termination for abnormality has financial implications. However, without the service women will continue to make decisions they later regret and which have a profound impact on their personal lives and their family as well as a potential extra demand on other services. Without an improvement in the waiting room in the ultrasound department women will continue to be given bad news and be left to digest the information with little privacy, which will contribute to their feeling of abandonment and alienation.

There are examples of when changes in the way the service is organised will improve care to women and where an increase in resources is not necessarily involved. In this hospital separating the care of women who miscarry from the acute services of the A&E department and the emergency ward would improve care for women. Restructuring follow-up care for women with second- and third-trimester pregnancy loss would not necessarily involve an increase in resources but would make more effective use of resources already available and could make a considerable difference to the women.

Even when organisational factors inhibit good care sensitive and committed individual professionals will be able, some of the time at least, to find ways around the system to reach women in the way they need even if the personal cost is high. Others will use the system as a valid excuse to avoid the more demanding aspects of care.

However, organisations can be structured to allow and encourage the professionals working within them to be more sensitive to the individuals for whom they are caring. A system that allows a personal relationship between a woman and her caregivers, that allows as far as possible continuity of care and that gives women more choice and some control will provide more sensitive care for women. The disjointed care that is provided for women who miscarry does not do this. The high-quality care offered by the midwives clearly does whereas the changes in carers that occur once a woman leaves hospital does not.

In addition to the system of care the qualities of the management are clearly important. The midwives feel supported by the management. The midwifery manager provides an excellent role model as a sensitive caregiver. The care the midwives are able to give is a reflection of the care they receive.

❑ Understanding women

Professionals' understanding of women is fundamental if care is to be made appropriate to the individual. A general understanding of the diversity of women's experiences of pregnancy loss and the broad-ranging impact it may have is essential. However, health professionals work under pressure and are faced with understanding women at a particular point in time. Most professionals do not have access to detailed background information about the woman. Only those who are likely to have long-term involvement with a woman, like some GPs, may have the opportunity to gain a full history. Moreover, many women would not wish to give this information and others would be unable to do so. Some women are inarticulate, particularly when faced with the crisis of a miscarriage, stillbirth or termination, and others will find it hard to trust professionals and to enter a relationship with them.

Drawing on the experiences of the women and the health professionals in this study an appreciation of the following differences between women appear to be the most relevant and provide a framework to help the health professional to understand a woman's reactions and the care that may be most appropriate to her:

- *The meaning of the pregnancy:* the way in which the woman relates to her pregnancy, whether or not she defines the pregnancy as a baby, and the degree of attachment that she has developed.
- *Her personal qualities:* particularly her emotional expressiveness, how explicit, how assertive or passive, and how public or private she wishes to be, as well as her expectations of health care.
- *Her coping resources:* women will differ in the ways in which they cope in a crisis, in their inner resources and in the social support they have or need at the time. Conversely, they will differ in the difficulties they bring with them to the situation that may make the pregnancy loss more or less difficult for them.

❑ Professional behaviour/responsibility

Providing care that is responsive to women as individuals places a particular responsibility on professionals. Care can only be individualised if women are helped by practitioners who listen, accept and do not attempt to control or define personal experience. Professionals have to face the pain of the experiences and their own powerlessness. It requires a relationship of greater equality between professional and patient; the professional bringing his or her professional knowledge and skills and the patient her knowledge of herself. It also places a responsibility on the professionals for greater openness, to give of themselves and to learn from women. Maintaining this approach is a constant struggle when working within a relatively rigid system of care under the constraints of time and limited resources.

The following aspects of professional behaviour are particularly pertinent:

- *An openness to women's experiences.* Professionals need to be guided by and to learn from women. Staff must be able to listen, to enter into a woman's world, to be comfortable with saying, 'I don't know but I'll find out.'
- *Be human.* A more equal relationship between patient and professional is based on a recognition of the humanity of the professional. It is important that professionals relate to patients on a human level. It is appropriate for professionals to show their feelings as long as the professional's feelings do not dominate and get in the way of the professional responsibility for providing effective care. Patients should not have to take responsibility for looking after professionals.
- *Do not make assumptions, always ask and check things out.* Individualising care means that professionals cannot make assumptions. Professionals must recognise that they usually only see the tip of the iceberg. Without discussing it with the woman and checking her views they do not know what the woman is feeling or wants and therefore the sort of care that is appropriate. Professionals must ask if this or that is appropriate, if this is what the woman would like to know or if she would like this done.
- *Be proactive.* Professionals have a responsibility to reach out to women and establish a relationship. Professionals must be proactive, taking the initiative to provide information and checking out what a woman wants or does not want to know or to happen.
- *Recognise when women want the professionals to take over.* Individualising care also means being open to the fact that there will be occasions when, medical emergencies aside, women will want to relinquish control and professionals have to make decisions on their behalf, either because they are too distressed and are unable to participate or because they prefer other people to take the responsibility. The process of miscarriage, termination and stillbirth is normally distressing and women are dependent on others to care for them.
- *Facing the fear.* Making explicit the emotional nature of pregnancy loss means that the painfulness of the experience and the feelings aroused have to be faced. Professionals cannot avoid their own feelings of sadness, fear and abhorrence. Only by exploring their reactions so that they feel comfortable with their own response will professionals be able to help others.

❏ Equipping staff to provide individualised care

Individualising care for women places enormous demands on professional staff. The way in which professionals behave towards women is a reflection of the way in which they themselves are treated. If they work in an uncaring, rigid organisation that is indifferent to their needs this will be reflected in the quality of care they are able to provide. It is imperative that the needs of the staff who provide care for women in distressing situations are attended to.

Health professionals need adequate training. A broad understanding of the range of experience and of women's diverse reactions is essential. Knowledge about the system of care and particular procedures is also vital. Most notable in this study was the widespread ignorance of disposal practice along with the lack of accurate information, when care was compartmentalised, about what the next step in the chain of health care actually involved. For example, GPs referring women requesting a termination of pregnancy were unaware of the limitations of the hospital consultation; the SHOs were unaware that, after a miscarriage, women on the emergency ward rarely talked to nurses in any depth.

Regardless of profession all staff need good communication skills if they are to provide individualised care. This means not only the ability to impart complex and distressing information, often with little time, in a sensitive and clear manner so that it is readily understood, but also the ability to listen and to recognise the emotional content. There is ample evidence in this study of good communication in terms of imparting information and providing a clear explanation. Women felt that communication with professionals was poor when they believed they were not listened to, were not given the opportunity to give their views and had their feelings ignored.

The pattern of future health care which focuses on individual need is based on a partnership between patient and professional. Traditionally, many professionals have operated an expert model of health care. The approach must be to start where women are and to look at the skills that health professionals need to acquire to establish more equal relationships. Some senior staff in leadership positions may need training in partnership models of working.

Attention must also be paid to the need for support for staff. They need opportunities to talk about their own particular difficulties with the work, for example, for a midwife, handling a dead baby or, for an emergency ward nurse, talking with women who miscarry. Staff also need the opportunity to talk about particularly difficult events that occur. The registrar who felt responsible for increasing Sue's suffering by failing to seriously consider a caesarean section and the registrar who eventually delivered her baby and feared the baby would be decapitated in the process are unlikely to forget the experience or the feelings it engendered in them. Neither have had the opportunity to process the impact of caring for this woman beyond thinking about it themselves, sharing the experience with their partner or a personal friend and cursorily mentioning it to their consultant. We can only speculate on the effect this will have on them and how they will behave when they encounter a similar situation in the future. It is likely that they will block it out, deny the reality or avoid the situation in some way, which will impinge on the quality of care they are able to provide.

The current provision of support does not go far enough. Support for professionals must be informed by an understanding of the detection and process of trauma. A support system must be integrated into the organisation in order to be effective; otherwise staff who use it will feel marginalised or stigmatised and those most in need may not take it up. A support system must respond to particular distressing events as they occur as well as to the more routine. It also must provide regular opportunities for staff to reflect on the personal impact of the work and to reconsider the ways in which they cope.

Although creating a sympathetic culture in which support between colleagues can be maximised is essential, informal, peer support alone is insufficient. To feel that immediate colleagues care and understand is important but peer support may not be the best way to resolve problems that arise and may result in merely passing round the problem. Whilst the open door policy and peer support operating for nursing and midwifery staff in this hospital were experienced positively they are no substitute for a more formalised routine system. Staff will not always ask for support when they need it. The support for doctors was woefully inadequate. Beyond a quick chat with a colleague, either a senior or a peer, there is no mechanism for doctors, whatever their level of experience, to gain professional support in this emotionally complex work.

■ Conclusion: breaking the rules, changing the rules

Professionals in free discussion about providing good care for women undergoing pregnancy loss often talk about 'breaking the rules'. What they mean by this is that the only way to do what they consider right for a particular individual is to break prescribed patterns of behaviour and do what they are not supposed to do, putting them at risk of being criticised by those in authority. The organisation of health care is rigid, inflexible and rule-bound, and professional patterns of behaviour often institutionalised, making it hard for professionals who wish to respond to individuals to do so.

Working in such an environment it is understandable why those sensitive to individual experience feel they must break the rules but if good care appropriate to individual need is to be provided the rules must not be broken but changed. The focus must move towards accepting individual experience and need, giving the emotional needs of patients and professionals a higher priority and encouraging and facilitating the relationship between patient and professional. The challenge then becomes how to maintain an individualised approach to care without its becoming institutionalised and losing effectiveness.

■ Suggestions for further reading

Burnard, P. (1992) *Communicate: A Communication Skills Guide for Health Care Workers*, London, Edward Arnold.

Dainow, S. and Bailey, C. (1988) *Developing Skills with People: Training for Person to Person Client Contact*, Chichester, John Wiley.

Graham, S.B. (1991) When babies die: death and the education of obstetrical residents, *Medical teacher*, 13(2):171–5.

Johns, C. (1995) Framing learning through reflection within Carper's fundamental ways of knowing in nursing, *Journal of Advanced Nursing*, 22:226–34.

Menzies, I.E.P. (1970) *The Functioning of Social Systems as a Defence Against Anxiety*, London, Tavistock.

Stewart, M., Bell Brown, J., Wayne-Weston, W. *et al.* (1995) *Patient-centred Medicine, Transforming the Clinical Method*, London, Sage.

Walter, T. (1994) *The Revival of Death*, London, Routledge.

Walter, T. (1996) A new model of grief: bereavement and biography, *Mortality* 1(1):7–25.

Appendix I

The research study

■ Purpose

The purpose of the project was to assist health professionals to improve professional practice across the spectrum of pregnancy loss. The experience of pregnancy loss from the perspectives of the women themselves and the professionals who cared for them was investigated with a view to describing good practice and identifying professional needs. The specific aims of the project were to:

- increase understanding of women's experiences of stillbirth, miscarriage and termination of pregnancy, and the health care that is helpful to them
- investigate the professional response to pregnancy loss in order to discover underlying attitudes, understanding and knowledge
- develop a framework to help health professionals understand a woman's reactions and the care that may be most appropriate for her
- identify the obstacles that prevent health professionals providing good care and strategies for improving professional practice.

■ Design of the study

The focus of interest is the interface between the woman and the professional but in the context of the health care system. It was important to access the subjective experience of all the participants to enable the reader to understand and enter the worlds of both the woman as patient and the professionals caring for her. It was also essential to understand the context of this experience, to understand the system of care and the way in which this defines the health care provided. To achieve this an in-depth case study approach was adopted. The study was based in one hospital so that detailed knowledge of the procedures and systems operating within this hospital could be gained. Within this context a series of cases of individual women and the health professionals who cared for them formed the focus of the study.

Stillbirth, miscarriage and termination at both early and late gestations were included in the study. Boundaries between the categories of experience based on gestation are often arbitrary and do not reflect women's experi-

231

ences. The contrast between voluntary and non-voluntary loss may not be as marked as might be expected. Some procedures are common across the experiences but are defined in different ways. For example, the arrangements for the disposal of the remains of a pregnancy after a miscarriage and after early termination of pregnancy are often not the same. Many health professionals have to deal with the range of experience. It was anticipated that comparison of health care for miscarriage, stillbirth and termination of pregnancy would yield insights into the social meaning attributed to the different experiences and reveal inconsistencies in care.

Pregnancy loss is a sensitive and emotional subject likely to arouse feelings in the women, in the professionals caring for them and in the researchers. These feelings are part of the focus of the research. Pregnancy loss is often a hidden experience and considered unacceptable to discuss. Only by gentle questioning and probing can these things be revealed and articulated. In addition feelings may get in the way of understanding some of the aspects of care. For example, facing up to the reality of an abnormal baby delivered in the second trimester is painful; thinking about how that baby is disposed of may be muddled by the feelings engendered. It is therefore important that the way in which the research is structured allows for the feelings of those under investigation to be acknowledged and explored. The researchers also need space, in the form of supervision and outside consultation, to deal with their own reactions.

The emotional nature of the research has to be taken into account when deciding on the most appropriate research methods to use. Failure to attend to this would limit the research findings. So the sensitivity of the subject matter, the desire to gain information about subjective experience and process and the need to understand a wide range of different but linked events dictated the nature of the methods adopted. Qualitiative research methods using semistructured interviews which allowed the participants in the research to explore the feelings aroused by the nature of the subject under investigation was therefore chosen.

■ Location of the study

A large provincial district general hospital was chosen for the research. It serves a population of approximately 200,000 in a largely urban area with a rural hinterland. The hospital is recognised in the locality as providing a high standard of care. The hospital was not chosen for this study because the standard of obstetric and gynaecological care was thought to be particularly poor and in need of review or because it was thought to be particularly progressive. The senior managers and practitioners were not defensive and were willing to participate in the study. They were open to improving their own practice and to reflecting on the changing practice in pregnancy loss and the dilemmas that any hospital faces in providing a high standard of care.

■ The research data

The research is based on three sources of local data:

- a review of the local service
- interviews with women experiencing pregnancy loss
- interviews with the health professionals who cared for them.

❏ Review of the local service

An overview of the service involved in the care of the pregnant woman and her dead baby was undertaken. The different sites, facilities and personnel were identified, including those departments which do not have direct patient contact (e.g. the histology laboratory) and are therefore not represented in our sample of health professionals but they nevertheless play a vital part in the service. Sites include the A&D department, the emergency ward, the gynaecology ward, the day surgery unit, two outpatient departments, the antenatal clinic and the midwifery unit. Other services are counselling, registration, pathology, mortuary and portering. Visiting the sites and talking to key managers and personnel has informed the interviews of both women and professionals. Copies of available procedures, protocols and information given to patients were obtained.

Beyond the hospitals there is a voluntary sector that offers support and information to women with unwanted pregnancies and following miscarriage, termination for abnormality and stillbirth. Information has been collected about the nature of each of the local voluntary organisations. There is also a privately run abortion clinic which has a contract with the health authority but which is not sampled by the study. Both the branch and clinic were visited and are a major resource for local women.

The different care routes for women through the system were identified. These are not always the same. For example, whilst women who miscarry in the first trimester are normally admitted to the emergency ward they may, in some circumstances, be admitted to the day surgery unit or the gynaecology ward.

❏ The sample

The women

The purpose of the project is to embrace the diversity of pregnancy loss and to understand the issues that confront health professionals caring for women within the system of care. The sample of women therefore does not aim to represent statistically the workload of the hospital but to reflect the range of women's experiences of the different categories of pregnancy loss.

Twenty women were recruited to the study between mid April and the end of June 1994. Details of the sample are given in Table A.1. The sample comprised:

- eight women whose pregnancy ended in stillbirth, mid-trimester miscarriage or termination
- six women who miscarried in the first trimester
- six women whose pregnancy was terminated in the first trimester, one for reasons of abnormality and five for other reasons.

Apart from the women having an early termination of pregnancy the women were contacted whilst in hospital and given information about the project. Pregnancy loss in the second and third trimesters is less frequent therefore, unless there was good reason not to, attempts were made to approach all the women in the hospital experiencing stillbirth, late miscarriage or late termination. The women were asked by their midwife if they would consider being involved in the project and would meet the researcher. None declined. Two women were missed because they were discharged from hospital earlier than expected and one woman was not approached because of the sensitivity of her case.

Table A.1   The sample: women

	Estimated occurrence	Women approached	In sample
Maternity unit			
stillbirth	6	4	3
late miscarriage	5	4	1
termination for abnormality	4	4	3
Emergency ward			
early miscarriage	55	9	6
termination (mid-trimester)	1	1	1
Day surgery unit			
termination (early)	109	7	5
Gynaecology ward			
termination for abnormality (early)	*	1	1
TOTAL		30	20

* Information not collected

NB: The occurrence is an estimate based on the regular collection of information directly from the different sites.

Early miscarriage and early termination were more frequent. Women were selected on a systematic basis to encompass the different medical teams and, according to the day of the week, to reflect possible differences in their care. Selection was made over a set period of time and ceased when the number for each category was reached. The women who miscarried were approached once sufficiently recovered from the ERPC. The researcher was briefly intoduced by a member of the nursing staff. None of the women declined to hear more about the project. The one woman admitted to the gynaecology ward for termination of pregnancy during the recruitment period for the study agreed to participate.

Women having an early termination of pregnancy were approached at the initial outpatient appointment and asked if they would be willing to join the study. Six outpatient clinics were attended. Of the 17 women attending appointments to request a termination of pregnancy seven agreed to talk to the researcher. One of these women was not willing to be contacted and another did not go ahead with the termination.

A couple of days after their discharge from hospital the women were telephoned at home to confirm their willingness or not to participate. In all, 30 women were approached. We have little information about those who refused to join the study. Of those who gave a reason the main theme seemed to be a reluctance to talk about their experience. As one woman said, 'I just want to put it behind me.' Three of the women were not at home in the week after their hospital admission and could not be contacted.

The women recruited to the study have a wide range of experience and reflect the variety of women cared for by the hospital. Their backgrounds and previous experiences of pregnancy are as varied as their response to the event. They vary from the well-educated, articulate graduate with a career to a woman who is barely literate and does temporary work as a packer in a factory; from women with close supportive relationships with their partner, family and friends to those who are very isolated and have hardly shared their experience; from women who are emotionally expressive to those who are more withdrawn and reserved. None of the 20 women systematically recruited to the study was from an ethnic minority. The hospital is in an area where approximately eight per cent of the population are from a variety of ethnic minority groups. More detailed background information about the women is given in Chapters 2, 3 and 4.

In order to place the sample of women in the context of the workload of the hospital it was necessary to establish the numbers involved in the different categories of loss. However, accurate figures about the incidence of pregnancy loss in the Trust were not easily obtained. The Trust collects its own statistics under two systems. At the time of the study the system was under review. Much of the information collected is aimed at measuring staff activity and not recording patient diagnosis. For example, the information on miscarriage is not easily identifiable; there are reasons other than miscarriage for an ERPC.

A ward-based tally of the numbers was conducted by the researchers for four months. This is recorded as the estimated occurrence in Table A.1. The numbers for second- and third-trimester pregnancy loss are small and the figures are likely to be accurate. Weekly figures were collected from the day surgery unit based on the theatre lists. The emergency ward was approached on a daily basis to record the women admitted that day. The staff initially gave the impression that the numbers of women admitted because of a miscarriage were much higher than the numbers we recorded.

The health professionals

At the first interview the women were asked to identify their GP; one woman did not wish her GP to be contacted. The women were then asked to identify four more health professionals who were significant in their care, either because they performed a key task or because they were particularly helpful or unhelpful. Selection was not based on the length of time of the contact – this varied – but on the significance of the contact to the woman. The women easily identified the health professionals on this basis.

Selecting the health professionals in this way was practical and also gave access to a wide range of health professionals with recent involvement in a case. Broad generalisations about the care that is usually provided for women in these circumstances, rather than focusing on what actually happens, could be avoided.

For the women interviewed later in the research there was occasionally a choice of health professional. For the sake of comprehensive coverage someone from an under-represented department or who had not been interviewed before was then selected. Table A.2 gives details of the sample of health professionals.

❏ The interviews

The interviews of both the women and the health professionals were based on semistructured interview schedules designed to elicit factors relevant to the research. The schedules were piloted and amended in the light of experience.

The aim of the schedules was to allow both the women and the health professionals to reflect on their experience of pregnancy loss and health care, with the maximum opportunity to say what had been important for them whilst at the same time ensuring that matters likely to be important, as shown by the research literature and the researcher's previous experience of similar research, were included.

The semistructured nature of the interviews allowed free interaction between the researcher and the interviewee and the opportunity to explore and uncover areas previously not considered. The researchers only pursued sensitive or difficult areas if there was a reason to do so and reminded the interviewee that questions did not have to be answered.

Table A.2   The sample: health professionals

	Professionals identified	Professionals interviewed
HOSPITAL STAFF		
Doctors:		
Obstetrician & Gynaecologists		
Consultant	8	4
Registrar	6	3
SHO	9	7
Anaesthetists		
Consultant	2	2
Registrar	1	1
SHO	1	0
Nurses:		
Emergency Ward		
Staff	7	5
Enrolled	1	1
Student	3	2
Antenatal Clinic		
Nursing Assistant	1	1
Main Theatre	2	1
Day surgery unit		
Sister	1	1
Staff	3	2
Enrolled	2	2
Gynaecology Ward		
Staff	2	2
Student	1	1
Outpateint Nurse	2	1
Midwives:		
Delivery Suite		
Sister	5	4
Staff	7	6
Postnatal Ward		
Sister	1	1
Staff	1	1
Sonographers	4	2
COMMUNITY STAFF		
GPS	19	15
Trainee	1	1
Practice Nurse	1	0
Community Midwives	4	3
Health Visitor	1	1
TOTAL	**96**	**70**

N.B.

1. All of the health professionals identified were approached. One of the health professionals was identified by four women, four of the health professionals were identified by three women and ten of the health professionals were identified by two women. In total 75 health professionals were approached.

2. Five women could only identify four health professionals. One woman identified two GPs and one woman did not want her GP approached.

3. Two GPs and the practice nurse were unable to participate.

4. An SHO and a student nurse moved to a new job before they could be interviewed.

The interviews were tape-recorded unless the interviewee refused permission (one woman) or, as with several of the health professionals, was brief. The tapes were used as an *aide mémoire*. Only sections of the tapes that illustrated particular points, were particularly insightful or were confusing and needed clarification were transcribed. Each of the researchers took responsibility for a selection of the different categories of cases but, by and large, interviewed the woman and all the health professionals connected with one case.

The women

The women were interviewed in their own home, the majority within a few days of their discharge from hospital. Three women were interviewed between seven and thirteen days after their discharge, one three weeks afterwards and another, who had initially refused to particiapte, a month afterwards. The interviews lasted about one and a half hours.

The interviews were handled with sensitivity, allowing the woman to dictate the pace of the interview and the order in which she discussed events. Attention was paid to the language the woman used to describe her experience, for example whether the word baby, fetus or embryo was used. The researcher picked up on the terms the woman used and noted any changes throughout the interview.

If a woman asked for help with specific issues it was discussed only in general terms. Suggestions were made of where she might get the information or help she required or alternative courses of action were discussed with her. Whilst it was hoped that the interview would be helpful to the woman by providing the opportunity for her to discuss her experience it was not the researcher's responsibility to provide specific help. The situation did not arise but, had the researchers been concerned about a woman's well-being, referral for further help would have been discussed with her. The researchers were professionally qualified as a community psychiatric nurse and social worker.

The women appeared to value the opportunity to share their experiences, some still actively grieving, others using the time to make sense of their experience or to re-tell a prepared story. They varied in the way they were able to reflect on their experience, some being able to answer only very direct questions or struggling to put words to their feelings, others being more articulate and needing few prompts.

It was planned to re-interview all the women approximately six months after their discharge from hospital. The second interview provided the opportunity to reflect on their experience as a whole but particularly their health care at the time and over the six month period. These too were taped and relevant sections transcribed. It was anticipated that the women's views about their health care might change over time and become more negative. The research did not bear this out. Some of the women's views intensified over time, that is, became more positive or more negative, but did not change dramatically.

In the intervening six months the researchers kept in touch with the women by means of a monthly diary sheet. This was to provide an ongoing and more accurate record of changes in the way the woman viewed her experience and her views of the health care she received and formed the basis of the second interview. It was made clear to the women that they could use the diary sheet as they wished, that the odd scribbled word was as acceptable as perfect prose.

Two of the women dropped out after the first interview because they moved out of the area; one had miscarried and the other had an early termination of pregnancy. Eighteen maintained contact over the six month period, usually by the monthly diary sheet or by telephone. One woman who was illiterate was visited regularly by the researcher. As anticipated the women varied in the way they used the diary sheet; several who wrote at great length said how useful it was whilst others wrote briefly and had to be reminded. Sixteen women agreed to the second interview. There is no available information on why the two women who had kept in touch in writing over the six months dropped out at this point. They may have felt that they did not want to rekindle memories of the miscarriage and termination.

The health professionals

The interviews with the health professionals normally took place within three weeks of the event and often much sooner. We were concerned that busy health professionals who may briefly encounter a large number of patients might not remember the woman recruited to the study but this was not a problem. Prompts of descriptions of the woman and the circumstances of the case were a sufficient reminder. Some of the GPs were interviewed later to allow for a longer period of contact with the woman.

The interviews varied in quality and in length from ten minutes to an hour and a half. This was only to be expected as, for some, the contact with the woman was fleeting and hard to recollect, so the focus of the interview was more general, whilst others had been involved in a more intense way or over a much longer period of time. With her permission issues identified by the woman about her health care were raised with the health professional. Where a staff member was identified for a second or third time a brief discussion or phone call about the case was sufficient.

The health professionals gave willingly of their time, either fitting us in to a busy work schedule or making time to see us when they were off duty. Many appear to have appreciated what may have been a rare opportunity to share their views and feelings about a potentially difficult area of their work and have done so with interest and in a spirit of openness and generosity.

■ Organisation and analysis of the data

All the interviews were analysed according to detailed schedules (data-recording sheets) covering the issues relevant to the research. In principle, and largely in practice, the interviews were collated under predetermined headings. Each interview would ideally have provided data for each of the headings of the schedule, although in practice some interviews provided more information on some topics than others. This enabled common themes to be drawn from the mass of interview material collected. The researchers worked separately and could provide an independent check on the conclusions drawn.

There are three aspects to the data analysis:

- health care
- professional needs
- ideas about pregnancy loss.

❑ Health care

Each case was analysed as a whole to incorporate the different perspectives of the women and health professionals and to identify the strengths and weaknesses of the women's care, as assessed against the views of the different participants, the accepted standards of good practice (the SANDS *Guidelines*) and the local system of care. This information was recorded on a case summary sheet. In addition different aspects of care were compared between cases. For this purpose the cases were grouped in the following way: the later losses to include stillbirth, mid-trimester miscarriage and termination (eight cases), first-trimester miscarriage (six cases) and first-trimester termination (six cases). This grouping reflects the different sites in the hospital where the women are cared for (the maternity unit, emergency ward or day surgery unit) as well as the different nature of the physical experience for women (labour and delivery or minor surgery).

❑ Professional needs

Themes in the health professionals' views on the personal impact of the work, support and supervision have been drawn out and compared and contrasted according to professional group and work setting. Attention was also paid to organisational issues, ideas about what constitutes good care and identifying the gaps in their knowledge and understanding of the service. This involved analysing the data under the following headings:

- personal impact of the work, including areas of special difficulty

- what they mean by support, what different models of support they experience, from whom they receive support, if at all, the particular issues on which they feel the need for support, and whether they value support
- what personal coping mechanisms they use to deal with the emotional impact of the work
- how well equipped they feel for doing the work, what preparation they have had for the different aspects of the work, and their views on their training needs
- their views on what constitutes good care
- their knowledge of the overall service provided to the women by the hospital
- the working relationships between the different professional groups
- the impact of the hospital organisation on how they are able to do their work as they would like.

❏ Ideas about pregnancy loss

Women's definitions of their experience have been drawn out from the interview data and compared with the legal and professional definitions. Health professionals' views of the different categories of pregnancy loss and the organisational definitions are also considered. This involved considering the data under the following headings:

- the ideas the women have about what to call their loss (for example was it a miscarriage, stillbirth or termination?)
- at what point do they define their fetus as a baby?
- how do these relate to the legal definitions and the views of the professionals?
- what models for understanding loss are used by the health professionals (for example gestation, voluntary and involuntary loss) and how do these match up with those of the women in their care?

By organising the material from the interviews in this way it has been possible to use the data to answer the questions that gave rise to this research project.

■ Confidentiality

It should be noted that the health professionals are not referred to by name but by their profession and status if that is relevant. The consultant obstetrician and gynaecologists are all referred to as he to protect the confidentiality of the one female consultant at this hospital. The women have all been given fictitious names.

■ Suggested further reading

Lee, R.M. (1993) *Doing Research on Sensitive Topics*, London, Sage.
Mason, J. (1996) *Qualitative Researching*, London, Sage.
Mays, N. and Pope, C. (1996) *Qualitative Research in Health Care*, London, BMJ.
Roberts, H. (ed.) (1992) *Women's Health Matters*, London, Routledge.

Appendix II
Useful addresses

British Association for Counselling
1 Regent Place, Rugby CV21 2PJ

Tel: (01788) 578328 (answer machine)

Information on where to get counselling locally. Send an A4 SAE.

British Pregnancy Advisory Service
Austy Manor, Wootton Wawen, Solihull, West Midlands B95 6BX

Tel: (0345) 304030 or (01564) 793225

Provides women who have an unwanted or unplanned pregnancy with professional support, information and advice and practical help under the terms of the 1967 Abortion Act.

Child Bereavement Trust
1, Millside, Riversdale, Bourne End, Bucks SL8 5EB

Tel: (01494) 765001

Training and support for professionals to enable them to address the needs of grieving families. Information for both professionals and bereaved families.

Cruse
Cruse House, 126 Sheen Road, Richmond, Surrey TW9 1UR

Helpline: 0181–332 7227
(Mon–Fri 9.30 am–5.00 pm)

Admin.: 0181–940 4818
(open 9.30–4.00 pm, closed 1–2 pm)

Support and advice for bereaved people.

Miscarriage Association
c/o Clayton Hospital, Northgate, Wakefield, West Yorks WF1 3JS

Tel: (019240) 200799 (9 am–4 pm Mon–Fri; out of hours answering machine gives alternative contact number)

Information and support for women and their families; publishes a newsletter and information leaflets; network of support groups and contacts throughout the country; will try to put women with similar experiences in touch with each other.

National Association of Bereavement Services
20 Norton Folgate, London E1 6DB

Tel: 0171–247 0617, (10 am–4 pm)
Counselling enquiries: 0171–247 1080
(10 am–4 pm and answerphone)

Counselling and support for anyone who is bereaved. Referral to a local bereavement service.

National Association for Staff Support
9, Carandon Close, Woking, Surrey GU21 3DU

Tel: (01483) 771599

Resources for professionals who wish to promote good support practices for health care staff.

National Childbirth Trust
Alexandra House, Oldham Terrace, Acton, London W3 6NH

Tel: 0181–992 8637 (9.30 am–4.30 pm)

Provides information and support for parents.

Perinatal Bereavement Unit
Tavistock Clinic, 120 Belsize Lane, London NW3 5BA

Tel: 0171–435 7111

A group of therapists with a special interest in late miscarriage, stillbirth and neonatal death. Available as a resource for practitioners and researchers. Can take some referrals (via GP) for women living in the London area.

Relate – National Marriage Guidance Council
Herbert Gray College, Little Church Street, Rugby, Warwickshire CV21 3AP

Tel: (01788) 573241 (9 am–5 pm), or see under Relate in the local phone directory

Offers help to couples or individual partners experiencing relationship difficulties.

Stillbirth and Neonatal Death Society (SANDS)
28 Portland Place, London W1N 4DE

*Tel: Admin.: 0171–436 7940
Helpline: 0171–436 5881*

Support for those whose baby dies after 24 weeks of pregnancy or in the early days of life. National network of support groups and contacts. Publishes newsletter and information leaflets.

Support Around Termination for Abnormality (SATFA)
73–75 Charlotte Street, London W1P 1LB

*Tel: Parents helpline: 0171–631 0285
Admin.: 0171–631 0280*

Support for parents through antenatal screening, testing and diagnosis of fetal abnormality. Training for health professionals to meet parents' needs. Publishes a range of literature for parents, families and professionals. National support network.

Twins and Multiple Births Association (TAMBA) Bereavement Support Groups
PO Box 30, Little Sutton, South Wirral L66 1TH

Tel: 0151–348 0020 (9 am–2 pm, answerphone after 2 pm)

For parents who have lost one or both twins, or babies from a multiple birth.

Women's Health and Reproductive Rights Information Centre (WHRRIC)
52 Featherstone Street, London EC1Y 8RT

Tel: information line 0171–251 6580 (10 am–4 pm, Mon, Weds, Thurs and Fri; answering machine out of hours)

Tel: Admin. line: 0171–251 6333

Information on most aspects of women's health and reproduction, publishes a quarterly newsletter and a range of information leaflets on particular topics. Reference library.

Bibliography

Abramsky, L. and Chapple, J. (eds) (1994) *Prenatal Diagnosis: The Human Side*, London, Chapman & Hall.

Adams, M. and Prince, J. (1990) Care of the grieving parent with special reference to stillbirth, in Alexander, J., Levy, V. and Roch, S. (eds), *Postnatal Care – A Research-based Approach*, Basingstoke, Macmillan.

Adler, N.E. (1992) Psychological factors in abortion, *Journal of American Psychology*, 47(10):1194–204.

Alexander, S. (1987) Grieving and caring – a student midwife's perception, *Midwives Chronicle*, 100(1195):240–2.

Alty, E. (1991) Miscarriage: creating support, *Nursing Times*, 87(2):22–3.

Appleby, L., Fox, H., Shaw, M. and Kuma, R. (1989) The psychiatrist in the obstetric unit: establishing a liaison service, *British Journal of Psychiatry*, 154:510–85.

Armsworth, M.W. (1991) Psychosocial response to abortion, *Journal of Counselling and Development*, 69(4):377–9.

Ashton, J.R. (1980) The psychological outcome of induced abortion, *British Journal of Obstetrics and Gynaecology*, 87:1115–22.

Ashurst, P. and Hall, Z. (1989) Motherhood thwarted: miscarriage, stillbirth and adoption, in Ashurst, P. and Hall, Z., *Understanding Women in Distress*, London, Tavistock/Routledge.

Baber, K.M. and Lunneborg P. (1993) Abortion – a positive decision, *Journal of Marriage and the Family*, 55(3):791.

Baluk, U. and O'Neill, P.O. (1980) Health professionals' perceptions of the psychological consequences of abortion, *American Journal of Community Psychology*, 8(1):65–75.

Bansen, S.S. and Stevens, H.A. (1992) Women's experiences of miscarriage in early pregnancy, *Journal of Nurse Midwifery*, 37(2):84–90.

Batcup, G., Clarke, J.P. and Purdie, D.W. (1988) Disposal arrangements for fetuses lost in the 2nd trimester, *British Journal of Obstetrics and Gynaecology*, 95:547–50.

Belsey, E.M., Greer H.S., Lal, S., Lewis, S.C. and Beard, R.W. (1977) Predictive factors in emotional response to abortion: King's termination study – IV, *Social Science and Medicine*, (2):71–82.

Berezin, N. (1982) *After a Loss in Pregnancy*, New York, Simon & Schuster.

Bluestein, D. and Rutledge, C.M. (1993) Family relationships and depressive symptoms preceding induced abortions, *Family Practice Resource Journal*, 13(2):149–56.

Blumberg, B.D. (1984) The emotional implications of prenatal diagnosis, in Emery, A.E.H. and Pullen, I.M. (eds), *Psychological aspects of genetic counselling*, London, Academic Press, pp. 202–17.

Bond, M. (1995) *Stress and Self Awareness: A Guide for Nurses*, Oxford, Butterworth Heineman.

Borg, S. and Lasker, J. (1982) *When Pregnancy Fails – Coping with Miscarriage, Stillbirth and Infant Death*, London, Routledge & Kegan Paul.

Bourne, S. (1968) The psychological effects of stillbirths on women and their doctors, *Journal of Royal College General Practitioners*, **16**:103–12.

Bourne, S. (1983) Psychological impact of stillbirth, *Practitioner*, **227**:53–60.

Bourne, S and Lewis, E. (1984) Pregnancy after stillbirth or neonatal death, *Lancet*, **289**:31–3.

Bourne, S. and Lewis, E. (1991) Perinatal bereavement: a milestone and some new dangers, *British Medical Journal*, **302**:1167–71.

Bourne, S. and Lewis, E. (1992) *Psychological Aspects of Stillbirth and Neonatal Death: An Annotated Bibliography*, London, Tavistock Clinic.

Brennan, M.D. and Caldwell, M. (1987) Dilatation and evacuation in the emergency department for miscarriage, *Journal of Emergency Nursing*, **13**(3):144–8.

Brewin, T. (1991) Three ways of telling bad news, *Lancet*, **337**:1207.

Bribing, G. (1959) Some considerations of the psychological processes in pregnancy, *Psychoanalytic Study of the Child*, **14**:113–21.

Burnard, P. (1992) *Communicate: A Communication Skills Guide for Health Care Workers*, London, Edward Arnold.

Butterworth, C. A. and Faugier, J. (1992) *Clinical Supervision and Mentorship in Nursing*, London, Chapman & Hall.

Byrne, J. (1992) Miscarriage study, *Journal of Science*, **257**(5068):310.

Callan, V.J. and Murray, J. (1989) The role of therapists in helping couples cope with stillbirth and newborn death, *Family Relations*, **38**(3):248–53.

Campbell, C. (1988) The impact of miscarriage on women and their families, *Nursing: Journal of Clinical Practice Education and Management*, **3**(32):11–14

Cancelmo, J.A., Hart, B., Herman, J.L. *et al.* (1992) Psychodynamic aspects of delayed abortion decisions, *British Journal of Medical Psychology*, **65**(Dec):333–45.

Carr, D. and Knupps, F. (1985) Grief and perinatal loss: a community hospital approach to support, *Journal of Obstetric, Gynaecological and Neonatal Nursing*, Mar/Apr:130–9.

Cecil, R. (1994) Miscarriage: women's views of care, *Journal of Reproductive and Infant Psychology*, **12**(1):21–9.

Cecil, R. (ed.) (1996) *The Anthropology of Pregnancy Loss*, Oxford, Berg.

Cecil, R. and Leslie, J.C. (1993) Early miscarriage: preliminary results from a study in Northern Ireland, *Journal of Reproductive Health*, **11**:89–95.

Chalmers, B. (1992) Terminology used in early pregnancy loss, *British Journal of Obstetrics and Gynaecology*, **99**:357–8.

Chalmers, B. and Meyer, D. (1992) A cross-cultural view of the emotional experience of miscarriages, *Journal of Psychosomatic Obstetrics and Gynaecology*, **13**:177–86.

Chervenak, F.A. and McCullough, L.B. (1990a) Clinical guides to preventing ethical conflicts between pregnant women and their physicians, *American Journal of Obstetrics and Gynecology*, **162**(2):303–7.

Chervenak, F.A. and McCullough, L.B. (1990b) Does obstetric ethics have any role in the obstetrician's response to the abortion controversy?, *American Journal of Obstetrics and Gynecology*, **163**(5–1):1425–9.

Chez, R.A., Davidson, G., Flood, B. and Lamb, J.M. (1982) Helping patients and doctors to cope with perinatal death, *Contemporary Obstetrics and Gynaecology*, **20**:98–134.

Clarke, M. and Williams, A.J. (1979) Depression in women after perinatal death, *Lancet*, (April 20):916–17.

Condon, J.T. (1986) Management of pathological grief reaction after stillbirth, *American Journal of Psychiatry*, **143**(8):987–92.

Condon, J.T. (1987) Prevention of emotional disability following stillbirth – the role of the obstetric team, *Australian and New Zealand Journal of Obstetrics and Gynaecology*, **27**(4):323–9.

Condon, J.T. (1993) The assessment of antenatal emotional attachment – development of a Questionnaire Instrument, *British Journal of Medical Psychology*, **66**(Jun):168–83.

Connolly, K.D. (1989) Factors affecting grief following pregnancy loss, in van Hall, E.V. and Everaerd, W. (eds), *The Free Woman: Women's Health in the 1990s*, Carnforth (UK), Parthenon.

Conway, K. (1991) Miscarriage, *Journal of Psychosomatic Obstetrics and Gynaecology*, **12**:121–31.

Cordle C.J. and Prettyman R.J. (1994) A 2-year follow-up of women who have experienced early miscarriage, *Journal of Reproductive and Infant Psychology*, **12**(1):37–43.

Cormell, M. (1990) Miscarriage, Unpublished dissertation, University of Surrey.

Cormell, M. (1992) Midwifery. Just another miscarriage?, *Nursing Times*, **88**(48):41–3.

Corney, R.T. and Horton, F.T. (1974) Pathological grief following spontaneous abortion, *American Journal of Psychology*, **131**:825–7.

Covington, S.N. and Theut, S.K. (1993) Reactions to perinatal loss: a qualitative analysis of the national maternal and infant health survey, *American Journal of Orthopsychiatry*, **63**(2):215–22.

Cranley, M.S. (1981) Development of a tool for the measurement of maternal attachment during pregnancy, *Nursing Research*, **30**(5):281–4.

Cuisinier, M.C., Kuijpers, J.C., Hoojduin, C.A.L. *et al.* (1993) Miscarriage and stillbirth: time since the loss, grief intensity and satisfaction with care, *European Journal of Obstetric Gynecology and Reproductive Biology*, **52**(3):163–8.

Dagg, P.K.B. (1991) The psychological sequelae of therapeutic abortion – denied and completed, *American Journal of Psychiatry*, **148**(5):575–85.

Dainow, S. and Bailey, C. (1988) *Developing Skills with People: Training for Person to Person Client Contact*, Chichester, John Wiley.

Dans, P.E. (1992a) Reproductive technology: drawing the line, *Obstetrics and Gynaecology*, **79**:191–5.

Dans, P.E. (1992b) Medical students and abortion: reconciling personal beliefs and professional roles at one medical school, *Academic Medicine*, **67**(3):207–11.

Danville, J. (1983) Helping the parents of a stillborn child, *Midwives Chronicle and Nursing Notes*, **96**(1148):308–10.

Davies, V. (1991) *Abortion and Afterwards*, Bath, Ashgrove Press.

Davis, D.L., Stewart, M. and Harmon, R.J. (1988) Perinatal loss: providing emotional support for bereaved parents, *Birth*, **15**(4):242–6.

Day, R.D. and Hooks, D. (1987) Miscarriage – a special type of family crisis, *Family Relations*, **36**(3):305–10.

Defrain, J. (1991) Learning about grief from normal families: SIDS, stillbirth and miscarriage, *Journal of Mental and Family Therapy*, **17**(3):215–32.

Defrain, J., Martens, L., Stork, J. and Stork, W. (1990) The psychological effects of a stillbirth on surviving family members, *Omega – Journal of Death and Dying*, **22**(2):81–108.

Department of Health (1991a) *Disposal of Fetal Tissue*, HSG(91):19, NHS Management Executive.

Department of Health (1991b) *Sensitive Disposal of the Dead Fetus and Fetal Tissue*. EL(91):144, NHS Management Executive.

Department of Health (1993a) *Changing Childbirth: Part 1. Report of the Expert Maternity Group*, London, HMSO.

Department of Health (1993b) *Changing Childbirth: Part 2. Survey of Good Communications Practice in Maternity Services*, London, HMSO.

De Vries, R.G. (1981) Birth and death: social construction at the poles of existence, *Social Forces*, **59**(4):1074–93.

Dunlop, J.L. (1979) Bereavement reaction following stillbirth, *Practitioner*, **222**:115–18.

Dunn, D.S. and Goldbach, K.R.C. (1991) Explaining pregnancy loss: parents and physicians attributions, *Omega – Journal of Death and Dying*, **23**:13–23.

Elder, S.H. and Laurence, K.M. (1991) The impact of supportive intervention after second trimester termination of pregnancy for fetal abnormality, *Prenatal Diagnosis*, **11**(1):47–54.

Englebardt, S.P. and Evans, M.L. (1988) Meeting consumer needs: successful collaboration between an interdisciplinary health care team and bereaved parents, *Nursing Connections*, **1**(1):57–63.

Estok, P. and Lehman, A. (1983) Perinatal death: grief support for families, *Birth*, **10**(1):17– 25.

Evans, M.I., Drugan, A., Bottoms, S. F., Platt, L.D. *et al.* (1991) Attitudes on the ethics of abortion, sex selection and selective pregnancy termination among health care professionals, ethicists and clergy likely to encounter such situations, *American Journal of Obstetrics and Gynecology*, **164**(4):1092–9.

Falek, A. (1984) Sequential aspects of coping and other issues in decision making in genetic counselling, in Emery, A.E.H. and Pullen, I.M. (eds), *Psychological Aspects of Genetic Counselling*, London, Academic Press, pp. 23–36.

Fewster, C. (1990) Death of a dream, *Community Outlook*, July:44–5.

Forrest, G. (1989) Care of the bereaved, in Enkin, M., Keirse, M. and Chalmers, I., *A Guide to Effective Care in Pregnancy and Childbirth*, Oxford, Oxford University Press.

Forrest, G.C., Claridge, R.S. and Baum, J.D. (1981) Practical management of perinatal death, *British Medical Journal*, **282**:31–2.

Forrest, G.C., Standish, E. and Baum, J.D. (1982) Support after perinatal death: a study of support and counselling after perinatal bereavement, *British Medical Journal*, **285**:1475–9.

Friedman, T. (1989) Women's perceptions of general practice management of miscarriage, *Journal of Royal College of General Practitioners*, **328**:456–8.

Friedman, T. and Gath, D. (1989) The psychiatric consequences of spontaneous abortion, *British Journal of Psychiatry*, **155**:810–13.

Gameau, B. (1993) Termination of pregnancy: development of a high-risk screening and counselling program, *Social Work in Health Care*, **18**(3/4):179–91.

Gannon, K. (1994) Psychological factors in the aetiology and treatment of recurrent miscarriage. A review and critique, *Journal of Reproductive and Infant Psychology*, **12**(1):55–64.

Garel, M., Blondell, B., Lelong, N. and Kaminski, B. (1993) Depressive disorders after a spontaneous abortion, *American Journal of Obstetrics and Gynecology*, **3**:1005.

Gaze, H. (1990) Making time to talk, *Nursing Times*, **28**(13):38–9.

Gilling-Smith, C., Toozs-Hobson, P., Potts, D.J., Touquet, R. and Beard, R.W. (1994) Management of bleeding in early pregnancy in accident and emergency departments, *British Medical Journal*, **309**:574–5.

Goldbach, K.R.C., Dunn, D.S. and Toedter, L.J. (1991) The effects of gestational age and gender on grief after pregnancy loss, *American Journal of Orthopsychiatry*, **61**(3):461–7.

Goldstein, S.R. (1990) Early pregnancy failure, *American Journal of Obstetrics and Gynecology*, **163**(3):1093.

Goodman, M. and Wigley, B. (1993) After miscarriage, *Health Service Journal*, **29**:29.

Goodwin, S. 1983) Caring for the carers. Part 2: Coping with stress, *Health Visitor*, **56**:46–7.

Gould, D. (1985) Understanding emotional need, *Nursing Mirror*, **160**(1):ii–vi.

Gould, P.T. (1992) The loss of a dream. Perinatal loss or an unexpected pregnancy outcome, *Journal of Perinatology* (US), **12**(3):262–5.

Graham, S.B. (1991) When babies die: death and the education of obstetrical residents, *Medical Teacher*, **13**(2):171–5.

Graves, W.L. (1987) Psychological aspects of spontaneous abortion in Bennett, M.J. and Edmonds, D.K., (eds), *Spontaneous and Recurrent Abortion*, Oxford, Blackwell Scientific.

Greer, H.S., Lal, S., Lewis, S.C. *et al.* (1976) Psychological consequences of therapeutic abortion. King's termination study III, *British Journal of Psychiatry*, **128**:74–9.

Hall, M.H. (1990) Changes to the abortion law, *British Medical Journal*, **301**:1109–10.

Hall, M.H. (1991) The health of pregnant women, *British Medical Journal*, **303**:460–2.

Hall, R.C.W., Beresford, T.P. and Quinones, J.E. (1987) Grief following spontaneous abortion, *Psychiatric Clinics of North America*, **10**:405–20.

Hamilton, M. (1989) Should follow-up be provided after miscarriage?, *British Journal of Obstetrics and Gynaecology*, **96**:743–5.

Harris, B.G., Sandelowski, M. and Holditch-Davis, D. (1991) Infertility... and new interpretations of pregnancy loss, *American Journal of Maternal Child Nursing*, **16**(4):217–20.

Hartman, A. (1991) Toward a redefinition and contextualization of the abortion issue, *Social Work*, **36**(6):467–8.

Harvey, P. (1983) You are saying goodbye to someone you have never said hallo to, *Community Care*, Nov 24:24–5.

Hawkins, P. and Shoet, R. (1989) *Supervision in the Helping Professions*, Milton Keynes, Open University Press.

Heimler, A. (1990) Group counselling for couples who have terminated a pregnancy following prenatal diagnosis, *Birth Defects*, **26**(3):161–7.

Henshaw, R.C., Cooper, K., El-Refael, H.L., Smith, N.C. *et al.* (1993a) Medical management of miscarriage: non-complete surgical uterine evacuation of incomplete and inevitable spontaneous abortion, *British Medical Journal*, **306**:894–5.

Henshaw, R.C., Naji, S.A., Russell, I.T. and Templeton, A.A. (1993b) Comparison of medical abortion with surgical vacuum aspiration: women's preferences and acceptability of treatment, *British Medical Journal*, **307**(6906):714–7.

Herz, E. (1983) Psychological repercussions of pregnancy loss, in Dennerstein, L. and de Senarclens, M. (eds), *The Young Woman: Psychosomatic Aspects of Obstetrics and Gynaecology*, Amsterdam, Excerpta Medica.

Hey, V., Itzin, C., Saunders, L. and Speakman M.A. (eds) (1989) *Hidden Loss: Miscarriage and Ectopic Pregnancy*, London, The Women's Press.

Hill, S. (1989) *Family*, London, Michael Joseph.

Hindmarch, C. (1994) *On the Death of a Child*, Abingdon, Radcliffe Medical Press.

HMSO (1992a) *Maternity Services Second Report of the Health Committee*. House of Commons Paper 29 1–3 Session 1991–1992, London, HMSO.

HMSO (1992b) *Government Response to the Second Report from the Health Committee*, Session 1991–92, Cm 2018, London, HMSO.

Hughes, P. (1987) The management of bereaved mothers: what is best?, *Midwives Chronicle*, **100**(1195):226–9.

Hulme, H. (1983) Therapeutic abortion and nursing care, *Nursing Times*, October:54–60.

Hunfield, J.A., Wladimiroff, J.W. and Passchier, J. (1993) Reliability and validity of the Perinatal Grief Scale for women who experienced late pregnancy loss, *British Journal of Medical Psychology*, **66**(3):295–8.

Hunt, S. (1984) Pastoral care and miscarriage: a ministry long neglected, *Pastoral Psychology*, **32**(4):265–78.

Hutti, M.H. (1984) An examination of perinatal death literature: implications for nursing practice and research, *Health Care for Women International*, 5(5–6):387–400.

Hutti, M.H. (1986) An exploratory study of the miscarriage experience, *Health Care for Women International*, 7:371–89.

Hutti, M.H. (1988a) Miscarriage: the parents point of view, *Journal of Emergency Nursing*, 14(6):367–8.

Hutti, M.H. (1988b) Perinatal loss: assisting parents to cope, *Journal of Emergency Nursing*, 14(6):338–41.

Hutti, M.H. (1988c) A quick reference table of intervention to assist families to cope with pregnancy loss or neonatal death, *Birth*, 15(1):33–5.

Iles, S. (1989) The loss of early pregnancy, *Baillière's Clinical Obstetrics and Gynaecology*, 3(4):769–90.

Iles, S. and Gath, D. (1993) Psychiatric outcome of termination of pregnancy for fetal abnormality, *Psychological Medicine*, 23(2):407–13.

Iskander, R. (1991) Perinatal bereavement, *British Medical Journal*, 303:122 (letter).

Jackman, C., McGee, H.M. and Turner, M. (1991) The experience and psychological impact of early miscarriage, *Irish Journal of Psychology*, 12(2):108–20.

Jacob, S.R. (1993) An analysis of the concept of grief, *Journal of Advanced Nursing*, 18(11):1787–94.

Johns, C. (1995) Framing learning through reflection within Carper's fundamental ways of knowing in nursing, *Journal of Advanced Nursing*, 22:226–34.

Johnson, M. (1989) Did I begin?, *New Scientist*, 124:39–42.

Joint Committee for Hospital Chaplaincy (1987) *Miscarriage, Stillbirth & Neonatal Death: Guidelines in Pastoral Care for the Clergy*, London, Joint Committee for Hospital Chaplaincy.

Kaltreider, N.B., Goldsmith, S. and Margolis, A.J. (1979) The impact of mid-trimester abortion techniques on patients and staff, *American Journal of Obstetrics and Gynecology*, 135:235–8.

Karcher, H.L. (1992) German doctors struggle to keep 15 week fetus viable, *British Medical Journal*, 305:1047–8.

Kennell, M.D., Slyter, H. and Klaus, M.H. (1970) The mourning response of parents to the death of a newborn infant, *New England Journal of Medicine*, 283(7):344–9.

Kenny, C.B. 1993) Social influence and opinion on abortion, *Social Science Quarterly*, 74(3):560–74.

Kenyan, S. (1985) No grave, no photograph, no baby, *Nursing Mirror*, 161(3):521–7.

Kirk, E.P. (1984) Psychological effects and management of perinatal loss, *American Journal of Obstetrics and Gynecology*, 149(1):46–57.

Kirkley-Best, E. (1982) The forgotten grief: a review of the psychology of stillbirth, *American Journal of Orthopsychology*, 52(3):420–9.

Kitzinger, J. (1990) Recalling the pain, *Nursing Times*, 86(3):38–40.

Klaus, M.H. and Kennell M.D. (1976) *Maternal–Infant Bonding*, CV Mosby, St Louis.

Knowles, S. (1994) A passage through grief – the Western Australia Rural Pregnancy Loss Team, *British Medical Journal*, 309:1705–8.

Kohner, N. (1984) *Midwives and Stillbirth: A Report of a Joint Royal College of Midwives/Health Education Council Workshop*, London, RCM.

Kohner, N. (1992) *A Dignified Ending*, London, SANDS.

Kohner, N. (1994) *Clinical Supervision in Practice*, London, King's Fund.

Kohner, N. and Henley, A. (1991, rev. edn 1995) *When a Baby Dies*, London, Pandora Press/HarperCollins.

Kohner, N. and Leftwich, A. (1995) *Pregnancy Loss and the Death of a Baby. A Training Pack*, Cambridge, National Extension College.

Kovit, L. (1978) Babies as social products: the social determinants of classification, *Social Science and Medicine*, 12:347–51.

Koziol-McLain, J., Whitehill, C.S., Stephens, L. *et al.* (1992) An investigation of emergency department patients' perceptions of their miscarriage experience, *Journal of Emergency Nursing* (US), 18(6):501–4.

Kunins, H. and Rosenfield, A. (1991) Abortion: a legal and public health perspective, *Annual Review of Public Health*, 12:361–82

Lake, M.F., Jonson, T.M., Murphy, J. and Knuppel, R.A. (1987) Evaluation of a perinatal grief support team, *American Journal of Obstetrics and Gynecology*, 157(5):1203–6.

Lancet (1977) The abhorrence of stillbirth, *Lancet*, 1188–90 (editorial).

Lancet (1991a) Perinatal mortality rates – time for change?, *Lancet*, 337:331 (editorial).

Lancet (1991b) When is a fetus a dead baby, *Lancet*, 337:526 (editorial).

Lapple, M. (1989) Coping behaviour in women with miscarriage or spontaneous abortion and recurrent spontaneous abortion, *Psychotherapy, Psychosomatic Medical Psychology*, 39(9–10):348–55.

Lask, B. (1975) Short term psychiatric sequelae to therapeutic termination of pregnancy, *British Journal of Psychiatry*, 126:173–7.

Lasker, J.N. (1991) Acute versus chronic grief: the case of pregnancy loss, *American Journal of Orthopsychiatry*, 61(4):510–22.

Lasker, J.N. and Toedter, L.J. (1994) Satisfaction with hospital care and interventions after pregnancy loss, *Death Studies*, 18:41–64.

Law, R.F. (1989) Abortion debate, *British Medical Journal*, 299:916–17.

Layne, L.L. (1990) Motherhood lost: cultural dimensions of miscarriage and stillbirth in America, *Women and Health*, 16(3–4):69–98.

Lazarus, A. and Stern, R. (1986) Psychiatric aspects of pregnancy termination, *Clinical Obstetrics and Gynaecology*, 13(1):125–34.

Leask, R. (1991) Miscarriage: too common a story?, *Nursing Times*, 87(2):22–3.

Leff, P.T. (1987) Here I am, Ma: the emotional impact of pregnancy loss on parents and health care professionals, *Family Systems Medicine*, 5(1):105–14.

Leon, I.G. (1990) *When a Baby Dies: Pyschotherapy for Pregnancy and Newborn Loss*, Yale, Yale University Press.

Leon, I.G. (1992a) Perinatal loss: choreographing grief on the Obstetric Unit, *American Journal of Orthophsychiatry*, 62(1):7–8.

Leon, I.G. (1992b) Perinatal loss – A critique of current hospital practices, *Clinical Pediatrics*, 31(6):366–74.

Leon, I.G. (1992c) Providing versus packaging support for bereaved parents after perinatal loss, *Birth*, 19(2):89–91.

Leppert, P.C. and Pahlka, B.S. (1984) Grieving characteristices after spontaneous abortion: a management approach, *Journal of Obstetric Gynaecology*, 64(1):119–22.

Leroy, M. (1988) *Miscarriage*, Optima, Macdonald.

Leschot, N.J., Verjaal, M. and Treffers, P.E. (1982) Therapeutic abortion on genetic indication; a detailed follow-up study of 20 patients, *Journal of Psychosomatic Obstetrics and Gynecology*, 1:47–56.

Lewis, E. (1976) The management of stillbirth. Coping with unreality, *Lancet*, 2:612–20.

Lewis, E. (1979) Inhibition of mourning by pregnancy: psychology and management, *British Medical Journal*, 2:27–8.

Lewis, E. and Page, A. (1978) Failure to mourn a stillbirth: an overlooked catastrophe, *British Journal of Medical Psychology*, 51:237–41.

Lewis, H. (1979) Nothing was said sympathy-wise, *Social Work Today*, 10(45):12.

Lloyd, J. and Laurence, K.M. (1985) Sequelae and support after termination of pregnancy for fetal malformation, *British Medical Journal*, 290:907–9.

Lorenz, P.L. and Kuhn, H. (1989) Multidisciplinary term counselling for fetal anomalies, *American Journal of Obstetrics and Gynecology*, Aug:263–5.

Lovell, A. (1982) Mothers and babies in limbo, *Nursing Mirror*, **155**(18):53–4.

Lovell, A. (1983a) Women's reactions to late miscarriage, stillbirth and perinatal death, *Health Visitor*, **56**:325–7.

Lovell, A. (1983b) Some questions of identity: late miscarriage, stillbirth and perinatal loss, *Social Science and Medicine*, **17**(11):755–61.

Lovell, A. (1983c) *A Bereavement with a Difference: A Study of Late Miscarriage, Stillbirth and Perinatal Death*, Occasional Paper, London, South Bank Polytechnic.

Lumley, J. (1980) The image of the fetus in the first trimester, *Birth Family Journal*, **7**:5.

MacLean, M.A. and Cumming, G.P. (1993) Providing for women following miscarriage, *Scottish Medical Journal*, **38**(1):5–7.

Macrow, P. and Elstein, M. (1993) Managing miscarriage medically, *British Medical Journal*, **306**:876.

Madden, M.E. (1988) Internal and external attributions following miscarriage, *Journal of Social and Clinical Psychology*, **7**(2):113–21.

Mander, R. (1994) *Loss and Bereavement in Childbearing*, Oxford, Blackwell Scientific.

Menzies, I.E.P. (1970) *The Functioning of Social Systems as a Defence Against Anxiety*, London, Tavistock.

Mitchell, S. (1988) Stillbirth: a patient's perspective, *Practitioner*, **232**:1368–71.

Moohan, J., Gashe, R. and Cecil, R. (1994) The management of miscarriage: results from a survey at one hospital, *Journal of Reproductive and Infant Psychology*, **12**(1):17–19.

Morgan, B.M., Bulpitt, C.J., Clifton, P. and Lewis, P.J. (1984) The consumers' attitude to obstetric care, *British Journal of Obstetrics and Gynaecology*, **91**:624–8.

Morris, D. (1988a) Disposal arrangements for second trimester fetuses, *British Jouranl of Obstetrics and Gynaecology*, **95**:545–6.

Morris, D. (1988b) Management of perinatal bereavement, *Archives of Disease in Children*, **63**(Jul):870–2.

Moscarello, R. (1989) Perinatal bereavement support service: three year review, *Journal of Palliative Care*, **54**:12–18.

Moulder, C. (1990, rev. edn 1995) *Miscarriage: Women's Experiences and Needs*, London, Pandora Press/HarperCollins.

Moylan, D. and Jureidini, J. (1994) Pain tolerable and intolerable: consultations to two staff groups who work in the face of potentially fatal illness, in Erskine, A. and Judd, D. (eds), *The Imaginative Body: Psychodynamic Therapy in Health Care*, London, Whurr.

Muller, R.T. (1991) In defense of abortion: issues of pragmatism regarding the institutionalisation of killing, *Perspectives in Biological Medicine*, **34**(3):315–25.

Murray, J. and Callan, V. (1988) Predicting adjustment to perinatal death, *British Journal of Medical Psychology*, **61**:237–44.

Nash, K.L. (1987) It's still a baby!, *Midwives Chronicle and Nursing Notes*, May:123–5.

NASS (1992) *A Charter for Staff Support for Staff in the Health Care Services*. Available from National Association for Staff Support, 9 Carandon Close, Woking, Surrey, GU21 3DU. Tel: (01483) 771599.

Neugebauer, R. (1987) The psychiatric effects of miscarriage: research design and preliminary findings, in Cooper, B. (ed.), *Psychiatric Epidemiology: Progress and Prospects*, London, Croom Helm.

Neugebauer, R., Line, J., O'Connor, P. *et al.* (1992) Depressive symptoms in women six months after miscarriage, *American Journal of Obstetrics and Gynecology*, **166**(1):104–9.

Neustatter, A. and Newson, G. (1986) *Mixed Feelings: The Experience of Abortion*, London, Pluto Press.

Ney, P., Fung, T., Wickett, A.R. and Beaman-Dodd, C. (1994) The effects of pregnancy loss on women's health, *Journal of Social Science and Medicine,* 38(9):1193–200.

Nielson, S. and Hahlin, M. (1995) Expectant management of first-trimester spontaneous abortion, *Lancet,* 345:84–6.

Oakley, A., McPherson, A. and Roberts, H. (1984, rev. edn 1990) *Miscarriage,* Harmondsworth, Penguin.

Osofsky, J.D. and Osofsky, H.J. (1972) The psychological reaction of patients to legalised abortion, *American Journal of Orthopsychology,* 42(1):48.

Page, L. (1993) Changing childbirth, *Modern Midwife,* Nov/Dec:28–9.

Panuthos, C. and Romeo, C. (1984) *Ended Beginnings: Healing Childbearing Losses,* Massachusetts, Bergin & Garvey.

Pare

Parkes, C.M. (1972) *Bereavement. Studies of Grief in Adult Life,* London, Tavistock.

Parkes, C.M. (1985) Bereavement, *British Journal of Psychiatry,* 146:11–17.

Peppers, L.G. and Knapp, R.J. (1980a) Maternal reactions to involuntary fetal–infant death, *Psychiatry,* 43(2):155–9.

Peppers L.G. and Knapp, J. (1980b) *Motherhood and Mourning,* New York, Praeger.

Pines, D. (1990) Pregnancy, miscarriage and abortion: a psychoanalytic perspective, *International Journal of Psycho Analysis,* 71:301–7.

Piontelli, A. (1992) *From Fetus to Child: An Observational and Psychoanalytic Study,* New Library of Psychoanalysis 15, London: Tavistock/Routledge.

Polkinghorne, J. (1989) *Review of the Guidance on the Research Use of Fetuses and Fetal Material,* Cm 762, London, HMSO.

Potvin, L. (1989) Measuring grief: a short version of the perinatal grief scale, *Journal of Psychopathology and Behavioural Assessment,* 11:29–45.

Prettyman, R.J. and Cordle, C.J. (1992) Psychological aspects of miscarriage: attitudes of the primary health care team, *British Journal of General Practice,* 42:97–9.

Prettyman, R.J., Cordle, C.J. and Cook, G.D. (1993) A three month follow-up of psychological morbidity after early miscarriage, *British Journal of Medical Psychology,* 66:363–72.

Pridjian, G. and Moawad, A.H. (1989) Missed abortion: still appropriate terminology, *American Journal of Obstetrics and Gynecology,* 161(2):261–2.

Procter, E. (1985) Too young to live, *Nursing Mirror,* 160(20):31.

Rajan, L. (1992) 'Not just dreaming'. Parents mourning pregnancy loss, *Health Visitor,* 65(10):354–7.

Rajan, L. (1994) Social isolation and support in pregnancy loss, *Health Visitor,* 67(3):97–101.

Rajan, L. and Oakely, A. (1993) No pills for heartache: the importance of social support for women who suffer pregnancy loss, *Journal of Infant and Reproductive Psychology,* 11(2):75–87.

Rando, T.A. (ed.) 1986 *Parental Loss of a Child,* Illinois, Research Press.

Rantzen, E. (1983) Devalued death, *Times,* Nov 9, p. 13.

Raphael-Leff, J. (1991) *Psychological Processes of Childbearing,* London, Chapman & Hall.

Reinharz, S. (1987) The social psychology of a miscarriage: an application of symbolic interaction theory and method, in Deegan, M.J. and Hill, M.R. (eds), *Women and Symbolic Interaction,* London, Allen & Unwin.

Reinharz, S. (1988a) What's missing in miscarriage?, *Journal of Community Psychology,* 16:84–103.

Reinharz, S. (1988b) Controlling women's lives: a cross-cultural interpretation of miscarriage accounts, *Research in the Sociology of Health Care,* 7:3–37.

Roberts, H. (1990) A baby or the products of conception: lay and professional perspectives and miscarriage, in Hall, E.V. and Everaerd, W. (eds), *The Free Woman: Women's Health in the 1990s*, Proceedings of the International Congress of Psychosomatic Obstetrics and Gynaecology, Carnforth, Parthenon.

Roberts, H. (1991) Managing miscarriage: the management of the emotional sequence of miscarriage in training practices in the West of Scotland, *Family Practice*, 8(2):117–20.

Robinson, G.E., Stirzinger, R., Stewart, D.E. and Ralevski, E. (1994) Psychological reactions in women followed for 1 year after miscarriage, *Journal of Reproductive and Infant Psychology*, 12(1):31–6.

Rogers, J., Stoms, G. and Phifer, J. (1989) Psychological impact of abortion: methodological and outcome summary of empirical research between 1966–1988, *Health Care for Women International*, 10(4):347–76.

Rosenfeld, A. (1991) Residency training and abortion, *American Journal of Obstetrics and Gynecology*, 6(1):1686.

Rosenfeld, J.A. and Townsend, T. (1993) Doesn't everyone grieve in the abortion choice?, *Journal of Clinical Ethics*, 4(2):175–7.

Rothman, B.K. (1986) *The Tentative Pregnancy: Prenatal Diagnosis and the Future of Motherhood*, London, Pandora Press.

SANDS (1986) *Stillbirth and Neonatal Death*, London, SANDS.

SANDS (1991) *Guidelines for Professionals: Miscarriage, Stillbirth and Neonatal Death*, London, SANDS.

SANDS (1995) *Pregnancy Loss and the Death of a Baby: Guidelines for Professionals*, London, SANDS.

SATFA (1995) *A Handbook To Be Given to Parents when an Abnormality is Diagnosed in their Unborn Baby*, London, SATFA.

Schoett, J. (1996) The needs of midwives: managing stress and change, in Kroll, D. (ed.), *Midwifery Care for the Future: Meeting the Challenge*, Eastbourne, Baillière Tindall.

Schott, J. and Henley, A. (1996) *Culture, Religion and Childbearing in a Multiracial Society*, Oxford, Butterworth-Heinemann.

Scott, H.R. (1989) Pregnancy – a barrier to grieving?, *Midwives Chronicle and Nursing Notes*, 102:332–3.

Seibel, M. and Graves, W. (1980) The psychological implications of spontaneous abortion, *Journal of Reproductive Medicine*, 25(4):161–5.

Seller, M., Barnes, C., Ross, S. *et al.* (1993) Grief and mid-trimester fetal loss, *Prenatal Diagnosis*, ·13(5):341–8.

Sherrat, D.R. (1987) What do you say, *Midwives Chronicle*, 100(1195):235–6.

Shusterman, L.R. (1979) Predicting the psychological consequences of abortion, *Journal of Social Science and Medicine*, 13A:683–9.

Slade, P. (1994) Predicting the psychological impact of miscarriage, *Journal of Reproductive and Infant Psychology*, 12(1):5–16.

Slade, P. and Cecil, R. (1994) Understanding the experience and emotional consequences of miscarriage, *Journal of Reproductive and Infant Psychology*, 12(1):1–3 (editorial).

Smith, A.C. and Borgers, S.B. (1988–89) Parental grief response to perinatal death, *Omega – Journal of Death and Dying*, 19:203–14.

Smith, A.M. (1977) The abhorence of stillbirth, *Lancet*, June:1315.

Smith, L.F.P. (1993) Should we intervene in uncomplicated miscarriage?, *British Medical Journal*, 306:1540–1.

Smith, N.C. (1988) Epidemiology of spontaneous abortion, *Contemporary Reviews in Obstetrics and Gynaecology*, 1:43–8.

Speraw, S.R. (1994) The experience of miscarriage: how couples define quality in health care delivery, *Journal of Perinatology*, 14(3):208–15.

Stack, J.M. (1980) Spontaneous abortion and grieving, *American Family Physician*, 21(5):99–102.

Stack, J.M. (1984) The psychodynamics of spontaneous abortion, *American Journal of Orthopsychiatry*, 54(1):162–7, 27R.

Statham, H. and Green, J.M. (1994) The effects of miscarriage and other 'unsuccessful' pregnancies on feelings early in a subsequent pregnancy, *Journal of Reproductive and Infant Psychology*, 12(1):45–54.

Stewart A. and Dent, A. (1994) *At a Loss: Bereavement Care When a Baby Dies*, London, Baillière Tindall.

Stewart, M., Bell Brown, J., Wayne-Weston, W. *et al.* (1995) *Patient-centred Medicine, Transforming the Clinical Method*, London, Sage.

Stierman, E.D. (1987) Emotional aspects of perinatal death, *Baillière's Clinical Obstetrics and Gynaecology*, 30:352–61.

Stinson, K.M., Lasker, J.N., Lohmann, J. and Toedter, L. (1992) Parents grief following pregnancy loss – a comparison of mothers' and fathers' response, *Family Relations*, 41(2):218–23.

Stirtzinger, R. and Robinson, G.E. (1989) The psychological effects of spontaneous abortion, *Canadian Medical Association Journal*, 140:799–805.

Stroebe, M.S., Hansson, R.O. and Stroebe, W. (1993) Contemporary themes and controversies in bereavement research, in Stroebe, M.S., Stroebe, W. and Hansson, R.O. (eds), *Handbook of Bereavement – Theory, Research and Intervention*, Cambridge, Cambridge University Press.

Strong, C. (1992) An ethical framework for managing fetal anomalies in the third trimester, *Baillière's Clinical Obstetrics and Gynecology*, 35(4):792–802.

Swanson-Kauffman, K. (1983) The unborn one: a profile of the human experience of miscarriage, *Dissertation Abstracts International*, 45(1–13):128. (Unpublished doctoral dissertation, University of Colorado.)

Swanson-Kauffman, K. (1988) There should have been two: nursing care of parents, *Journal of Perinatal and Neonatal Nursing*, 2(2):78–86.

Symonds, J. (1988) The psychology of spontaneous abortion, *British Journal of Theatre Nursing*, 25:27–31.

Thapar, A.K. and Thapar, A. (1992) Psychological sequelae of miscarriage: a controlled study using the general health questionnaire and the hospital anxiety and depression scale, *British Journal of General Practice*, 42:94–6.

Thayer, B. *et al.* (1990) Development of a peer suport system for those who have chosen pregnancy termination after prenatal diagnosis of a fetal abnormality, *Birth Defects*, 26(3):149–56.

Thong, K.J., Dewar, M.H. and Baird, D.T. (1992) What do women want during medical abortion, *Contraception*, 46(5):435–42.

Thullen, J.D. (1977) When you can't cure, care, *Professional Nurse*, Nov–Dec, 31–46.

Todman, J.B. and Jauncey, L. (1987) Student and qualified midwives' attitudes to aspects of obstetric practice, *Journal of Advanced Nursing*, 12:49–55.

Toedter, L.J., Lasker, J.N. and Alhadeff, J.N. (1988) The perinatal grief scale: development and initial validation, *American Journal of Orthopsychiatry*, 58(3):435–49.

Tom-Johnson, C. (1990) Talking through grief, *Nursing Times*, 66(1):44–6.

Tunaley, J., Slade P. and Duncan, S.B. (1993) Cognitive processes in psychology adaptation to miscarriage: a preliminary report, *Psychology and Health*, 8:369–81.

Turner, M. (1989) Spontaneous miscarriage: this hidden grief, *Irish Medical Journal*, 82(4):145.

Turner, M.J. (1991a) The miscarriage clinic: an audit of the first year, *British Journal of Obstetrics and Gynaecology*, 98:306–8.

Turner, M.J. (1991b) Management after spontaneous miscarriage, *British Medical Journal*, **302**:909–10.

Urquhart, D.R. and Templeton, A.A. (1991) Psychiatric morbidity and acceptability following medical and surgical methods of induced abortion, *British Journal of Obstetrics and Gynaecology*, **98**:396–9.

Wall-Haas, C.L. (1985) Women's perceptions of first trimester spontaneous abortion, *Journal of Obstetric Gynecology and Neonatal Nursing*, **14**(1):50–3.

Walter, T. (1994) *The Revival of Death*, London, Routledge.

Walter, T. (1996) A new model of grief: bereavement and biography, *Mortality*, **1**(1):7–25.

Wathen, N.C. (1990) Perinatal bereavement, *British Journal of Obstetrics and Gynaecology*, **97**:759–61.

Weaver, R.H. and Crawley, M.S. (1983) An exploration of paternal–foetal attachment behaviour, *Nursing Research*, **32**:68–72.

Wells, C., Morgan, D. and Leat, D. (1991) Fetuses and burials, *New Law Journal*, **26**(Jul):1046–7.

White, V.M. (1994) The moral status of the fetus, *Midwives Chronicle and Nursing Notes*, **107**(1281):375–9.

White-van Mourik, M.C.A., Connor, J.M. and Ferguson Smith, M.A. (1990) Patient care before and after termination of pregnancy for neural tube defects, *Prenatal Diagnosis*, **10**:497–505.

White-van Mourik, M.C.A., Connor, J.M. and Ferguson Smith, M.A. (1992) The psycho-social sequelae of a second-trimester termination of pregnancy for fetal abnormality, *Prenatatal Diagnosis*, **12**(3):189–204.

Williamson, W. (1988) Miscarriage – sharing the grief, facing the pain, healing the wounds, *Issues in Perinatal Care and Education*, **15**(4):252–3.

Wolff, J.R., Nielson, P.E. and Schiller, P. (1970) The emotional reaction to a stillbirth, *American Journal of Obstetrics and Gynecology*, **108**(1):73–7.

Zaccardi, R., Abbott, J. and Koziol-McLain, J. (1993) Loss and grief reactions after spontaneous miscarriage in the emergency department, *Annals of Emergency Medicine* (US), **22**(5):799–804.

Zeanah, C.H., Dailey, J.V., Rosenblatt, M.J. and Satter, D.N. (1993) Do women grieve after terminating pregnancies for abnormalities?, *Obstetric Gynecology*, **82**(2):270–5.

Zlatnik, F. (1986) Management of fetal death, *Clinical Observation and Gynaecology*, **29**(2):220–9.

Zolese, G. and Blacker, C.V.R. (1992) The psychological complications of therapeutic abortion, *British Journal of Psychiatry*, **160**:742–9.

INDEX